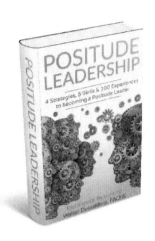

Dusseldorp & Associates, Inc.

107 Strawtown Road

New City, NY 10956

(646) 208-5217

www.positudeleadership.com

**ISBN-13:
978-1535325585**

**ISBN-10:
1535325585**

Positude Leadership

Four Strategies, Five Skills, and One Hundred Experiences

Walter Dusseldorp, MBA, FACHE

Positude leadership literally means leading with a positive attitude.

How is this strategy different from all the others? Simplicity in its meaning and implementation: simply be *awesome* every day!

This strategy is intended not only for hospital leadership. I wrote the book from my perspective as a hospital administrator and reference health-care management throughout; however, our strategies and skills are highly transferable to business management as well, regardless of industry.

Leading with great enthusiasm, passion, skill, knowledge, and ability in a mind-set of positive attitude—or *positude*—will most definitely enhance the likelihood of success in most business or health-care environments.

I challenge you, the reader, to become a *positude* leader.

Your commitment to positive leadership will lead to significant improvements in staff engagement and, ultimately, will lead to cost reduction, revenue increases, and increases in quantifiable safety and quality metrics.

Feel inspired; be inspiring!

You are awesome!

Special Acknowledgments

Behind every great book are many supporters.

I'm truly, deeply appreciative to the following folks for taking the time to provide honest feedback, critique my writing and design work, and assist me with putting the final touches on the first book in my *Positude* Leadership series:

My daughters: Abigail, Kimberlie, and Maia

My sons: Erik and Max

My best friends: Alex and Mark

My partners at Rockland Paramedic Medic 3: Bern, Shelly, and Joel

My mentors: Mark, Kirk, Lee, and Bob

My colleagues: Kevin, Will, and Jason

My wife, Erica, for putting up with the many hours I was glued to my Surface Pro 3, wondering what the hell I was doing

I would like to dedicate my first book to my guiding light, Martijn Tomassen. You are always on my mind.

Thank You

In life, you will come across many special people who will have a profound impact on your life. I have had the privilege to meet a few who have made a difference on my journey and would like to acknowledge them briefly.

Danny Klune—For teaching me a basic but powerful principle, to *relate* and not *compare*, which put me on a path of sobriety.

Michael Miksad—For trusting in my abilities as a young administrator, giving me room to grow, letting me learn from my mistakes, and expanding my role to gain more diversified experiences.

David Freed—For pushing me out of my comfort zone, which led me to explore new horizons.

Chris Fugazy—For pointing out that less is more, which is a constant reminder to practice my cadence to maximize effect. I'm deeply appreciative to you for allowing me to be creative and explore new ways to manage through *positude* leadership.

Mark Smith—For always being willing to listen, which allows me to decompress. An outsider would never understand our unique relationship, but it works.

Mark Oborn—For providing me with valuable insight and guidance on multiple levels of personal and professional development. I'm a better leader and person today because of your efforts.

Special Acknowledgments
What Is *Positude*?
Foreword—The Beginning, by Elizabeth Saviola, MS, OD
Preface
1. Creating Your Own Mini Culture
2. Four Strategies • Be Responsible…Love Those You Lead • Lead through Context • Ensure a Successful Environment • Use the Power of Focus
3. Five Essential Skills to *Positude* Leadership • Deep Listening • Apologize When Appropriate • Feedback • Developing a Common Bond • Make It a Safe Process
4. One Hundred Experiences
5. Is your Team a Team?
6. Finding the Right Teammates!
7. What Is Your Leadership Style?
8. Every Day Is a New Beginning
9. Reluctance to Change
10. What to Do If Your Project Fails
11. Gain Strength through Adversity
12. Are You Ready for a 360?
13. Man Down
14. *New Minute Manager*, a Quick, Powerful Read
15. Why Goal Setting Is Essential to Success
16. Do You Praise Enough?
17. How to Best Provide Redirection
18. Why Don't We Share Our Best Practices?
19. What to Do with Low Performers
20. What Works Best? Asking versus Telling
21. How to Recruit for Success

22. Do You Have an Active Rerecruit Strategy?
23. When Was the Last Time You Had Some Fun?
24. Why Team Building Is a Necessity!
25. Loving Those You Lead
26. Laser Focus
27. What to Do with Feedback
28. Meaningful Metrics—Do You Agree?
29. Driver Metrics—What Are They?
30. How Do Outcome Metrics Affect Us?
31. Crucial to Create Wins for the Team
32. Connecting the Dots
33. Staying on Top—Read a Lot?
34. Are You a Change Agent?
35. Transformation to Stay Ahead
36. Stagnation Will Lead to Disaster
37. How Do You Work with Unions?
38. Building Bridges between Key Stakeholders
39. Do You Have a Bully in the Workplace?
40. Are You Really Listening?
41. Are You Committed to Improving Every Day?
42. Everything We Do Is Just Another Process
43. Haunted by Policy
44. Regulations: Guardrail versus Guide Rail
45. Are We Still Allowed to Use Our Common Sense?
46. Risk Mitigation
47. Do You Know the Cost of Everything?
48. Complacency—Old versus New
49. It All Starts with Trust
50. Partnering with Adversaries
51. If It Were Only That Simple: Cut the Bottom 10 Percent
52. Does Culture Really Eat Strategy for Breakfast?
53. Only When You Change the Game
54. Are We Huddling Enough?
55. Is There Anything More Important Than Quality?

56. Political Capital: How to Spend Your PC Money
57. Can We Convert Naysayers?
58. Are You Really Committed?
59. Tolerance
60. Living in the Now
61. What to Do with a Saboteur
62. Ice-Cream Socials
63. Succession Planning—Are You Ready to Leave?
64. Good Ol' Boys' Club: Should I Join?
65. Fiscal Responsibility
66. Thank-You Cards—When Was the Last Time You Wrote One?
67. Walk Rounds: With Whom, Where, and When?
68. Physical Fitness: An Integral Piece of the Puzzle
69. Mental Fitness: An Absolute Must
70. Being Awesome
71. Why Mentoring Is Important to Personal Growth
72. How to Be a Great Mentee
73. Professional Associations—Should I Join?
74. Hiring: Passion, Skill, Knowledge, Ability
75. When to Let Go
76. Creativity over Capital
77. Labor Relations—Not Again
78. EQ—It's a Muscle
79. PQ—Positive Intelligence: Who Made This Up?
80. Is IQ Still Important?
81. What Is Your Behavioral Capacity?
82. Are You Accountable to Yourself?
83. Silence
84. Ask, Tell, Ask—Do You?
85. KISS—Keep It Simple, Stupid?
86. Networking for Professional Development
87. Paying It Forward—How/When/Why?
88. Checklist—Wheels Down
89. Leading Edge versus Trailing Edge

90. When to Pick Up the Phone versus E-mail
91. Creating a Safe Zone
92. Leading with Confident Humility
93. Why Be a Servant Leader?
94. Keeping a Scorecard
95. Are You on Track?
96. When to Say, "What?"
97. Patient Experience Should Come First
98. Should We Compare or Relate?
99. Team Concord—Do You Have It?
100. Personal Elevator Speech: You Have Thirty Seconds...Go!
101. Finding a Role Model
102. Learn from Others' Mistakes
103. Partnership Vital to Your Success
104. Closing the Deal
105. Conclusion
Appendix A: Recommended Reading List
Appendix B: Reference Materials
Appendix C: Tool Kit Expanded Exercises

What Is *Positude* Leadership?

Positive behaviors + right attitude + passion = *positude* leadership

Today, it's just not good enough to be just good enough; doing the right things in the right way has a whole new meaning in a health-care setting. Competition is fierce; every error or near miss is highlighted, and revenue is earned only through performance.

We need staff members who have the behavioral capacity, consistent passion, and delightful attitudes to make a lasting impression on our customers, both internal and external. Patients now have a choice, and they will vote with their feet if they are not satisfied with your services.

Great health-care institutions continuously reassess their positions in the marketplace and make adjustments, often on the fly, to stay ahead in an economic environment where shrinking budgets are the new norm.

As leaders, it is our responsibility to unlock employee's passion for excellent service and develop the right attitudes and positive behaviors to provide safety, quality, and satisfaction to our patients. It's difficult but meaningful work.

In about forty thousand words, you will learn—from my personal experiences, readings, conferences, and coaching and mentorships—ways to become a *positude* leader. As I once learned—and take this to heart—we need to *relate*; don't compare, and you will learn much.

Are you a *positude* leader in your hospital?

Foreword—The Beginning

by Elizabeth Saviola, MS, OD

Most of us have heard the empirical philosophy that people come in and out of our lives at certain times for certain reasons. If we are lucky, those connections stand out as special and unique and very often leave an indelible mark on our life experiences—personal and professional. We value those acquaintances and wonder how we got so lucky, how the stars were aligned, how the timing was right, how we were in the right place at the right time, how that "perchance" meeting opened a door, started a new chapter, launched a career, created an opportunity, altered a path, and leveraged transferable skills.

That galactic symmetry took me into its orbit not once but twice—first, early in my career, when I met Jack, who would become my mentor and friend. A kindred spirit ten years my senior, Jack was, like me, from a humble, challenging, inner-city upbringing yet confident in our shared values and life experiences, trust in the human spirit, and tough, street-smart determination to overcome the odds and succeed at being our personal best. Tasked with a corporate transformation, he was a game changer; he recruited me to his team, and I was all in. A decade apart, we both began our careers in clerical ranks and rose to the C-suite. I revel in my gratitude and *positude*, taking every opportunity to pay it forward by mentoring, coaching, and fostering teachability (hold that thought!).

My second "perchance" was meeting Walter, our author, a kindred spirit. We met when I was exploring new opportunities in health-care consulting, wanting to leverage my experience as corporate HR director with AT&T, VP of Electronic Services at Aetna, and national and international consulting in organization development—my lifelong passion and the root of all success in personal and professional life, because it gives us insight into how individuals, groups, teams, and organizations work: professional partnerships, personal relationships, and even families.

Squeezed into a one-hour slot on his prime-real-estate calendar, I was beyond thrilled that, in an unexpected hospital setting, Walter sounded like he was fresh from a Jackson Hole think-tank retreat, clearly articulating a vision for individual and organizational growth founded in physician leadership, team development, staff engagement, patient experience, and the ultimate: individual/team/organization *accountability*. Was this a *corporate* hospital?

I thought, *A tonic on a hot summer day, like finding a fluent English-speaking guide on a backcountry camping trip*. Here, where professional advancement is defined by credentialed medical education, clinical breakthrough, and industry-recognition designations, we talked about the void and the urgency of clinical leadership skills, the very basic, conspicuously absent, business/management mind-set, finishing each other's sentences in a rapid-fire, congruent cadence about core values, feedback techniques, rewards and recognition, open communications, mutual respect, team development, and on and on and on. What Walter saw and embraced as the challenges to solvency and competition and market share was that it is all about performance-driven goals and measurement, technical skills, and, yes, what often gets overlooked and underwhelmed—behavioral capacity (more on that later).

Walter was speaking the language of organization development. He understands the importance of knowing what makes us tick and tock; the impact of our experiences and beliefs; the drive of our stated and unstated wants and desires of leadership; the need to be heard, valued, and respected; the strength of our natural talents, skills, and abilities; and how all these dynamics are resident and at play among individuals, teams, and organizations, as well as how successful, star-quality leaders tap into those dynamics versus shying away from them, embracing the diversity of every characteristic and attribute of each individual to scream at the top of our lungs, "One plus one equals three!" He was talking about the need for a seismic culture change throughout the organization, daring to do things differently and with risk. A kindred spirit. A game changer. And I was all in.

And So We Began

A leadership framework, structured by teams, accountability, and professional development, guided the *positude* of this transformation and provided the victories, speed bumps, invaluable mistakes, lessons learned, and life-lasting ahas you will read about, thumb through, highlight, reference, and relate—not compare (you'll understand this later)—in the following pages.

Powered by an objective all-staff engagement survey, Walter established a baseline for change: communications, teamwork, leadership—all scored in the lower quadrants of a national scale. He engaged senior leadership in the discussion and solutions to what needed to change. Under a shared-governance model, Walter and the senior team appointed physicians, nurses, and administrative directors to team-lead positions—most were rookies—supporting them with tools, education, coaching, and mentoring in structured and flexible formats. Within fifteen months, twenty-two practice teams were formed; the original twelve teams completed fifty-nine projects in a twelve-month period. The ten new teams are in various stages of team development, but all are working within a ninety-day project cycle. Professional development for all teams and team members includes how-to, when-to training in communications, feedback, SMART goal setting, delegation, conflict resolution, and a repertoire of team-development skills. As a means of sustaining teachability, Walter instituted lunch 'n' learn leadership, a biweekly series of topics, lecturettes, and exercises, open to all hospital staff and designed to create awareness of individual, team, and organization strengths, insights, leadership, and communications style; relationship building; and creative solutions modeling.

KISS—there's more on this, but, yup, keep it simple. These big words translate to simple lessons, so if you're ready, flip the pages, and you will hear for yourself.

The business equivalent of taking Little League to the World Series, youth football to the Super Bowl, playground basketball to the NCAA finals, country-club tennis to the US Open, and high-school soccer to the World

Cup—OK, maybe a s-t-r-e-t-c-h, but you get the idea—this book will cover going from *good* to *great* with *a sense of urgency*.

You Got Talent!

Taking team members' natural talents and channeling them to one team concord, one common bond, and setting an expectation of accountability through weekly meetings, weekly metrics, and ninety-day projects—that's how it's done. Setting an expectation of professional development through self-awareness, stakeholder feedback, countermeasures, and action plans—that's how it's done. Setting an expectation of being a responsible leader through caring for those you lead and creating an environment of mutual respect and emotional safety—that's how it's done.

And That's How It's Done

And that's how Walter did it. You'll learn more about this in a great chapter: "Right People, Right Roles." He's the right person in the right role, and so is she; are you? *Yes!* And hearing the story of what Walter did and how he did it and his continuous learning and insights to be the change he wants to see—owning the idea that change begins with me—that's how it is done. And that's how you can do it!

There are numerous courses, webinars, textbooks, self-help books, and apps to help you become a leader. I have taken and taught and lectured and consulted on every permutation of leadership skills. By the time you've enjoyed your second cup of coffee or second glass of wine or registered online for a two-part adult-education leadership seminar, you could have saved fifteen minutes reading the strategies, skills, and stories of a *positude* game changer.

But leadership—at least *positude leadership*—is not easy, and it is not without personal and professional challenges. It means balancing the heart and mind, yours and others'; listening to both; and taking a risk with one over the other for the good of the individual, team, or organization. It means knowing yourself—the good, the bad, and the ugly—and embracing it all...in yourself and in others. It also means modeling your behavioral capacity, being confidently humble, apologizing appropriately, taking one for the team (like jumping in the lake and taking a dilapidated raft around a buoy so the team completes the exercise), or being vulnerable (like getting into the dunking booth at the staff BBQ so folks can see it's OK to have fun).

Sometimes, it means rowing out there alone to lead the way. I don't often quote *The Prince*, and I don't subscribe to Niccolò's leadership strategies, but I offer this passage as a sober afterthought to rising above the crowd, daring to challenge yourself, and putting into play the lessons for life on the next hundred pages:

It ought to be remembered that there is nothing more difficult to take in hand, more perilous to conduct, or more uncertain in its success, than to take the lead in the introduction of a new order of things. Because the innovator has for enemies all those who have done well under the old conditions, and lukewarm defenders in those who may do well under the new.
    —Niccolò Machiavelli, *The Prince*

Enjoy your journey, enjoy your life, and enjoy who you are about to become: a *positude* leader!

Lee Saviola, MS, OD

July 2016

Preface

One of my lifelong goals has been to write a book that not only tells a story but that, more importantly, allows others to learn from my experiences.

Each of us has something to offer to humanity; however, not many of us ever take the time to write down our own experiences. Nor are we likely to share commonsense solutions or best practices, even within our own four walls.

As you progress through my book, try not only to visualize the tasks you need to complete but to actually *do* them, even if it's with just a few staff members in mind.

These vital strategies and skills have elevated my performance from being a doer to managing, and now effectively leading, a large division of multiple disciplines in two very busy academic hospitals. It is an awesome feeling to see a group become a high-performance team. You, too, can accomplish this by being a *positude* leader who is passionate, nimble, and pragmatic and articulates a clear vision and collaboration in your transformational journey.

Are you teachable? Are you ready to learn? Are you ready to relate?

If you said yes to any of the above, you have come to the right place, and my hope is that you will walk away inspired and motivated to be the change you want to see. You are in charge of your future; come join me on a journey to learn from my mistakes, successes, and everything in between.

A Little Background

It would be very helpful to start with a short story about me.

Born in beautiful Delft, Holland, in 1970, just four pounds and a few ounces, I came into this world in a big rush. Six weeks early, I could wait no longer to meet my mom and dad. We settled in Zeddam, Holland, a small village not too far from the border of Germany. Within three and a half years, there were three of us kids; I was the only boy, born between my big sister, Judith, and my baby sister, Meta, both of whom frequently served as my personal punching bags—at least that's what they claim. I have no recollection of such behaviors.

Through my formative years, I was exposed to all the typical scrutiny every kid experience. I was bullied, and I bullied; I loved some and fought with others. One thing's for sure: my life was not boring for a single minute.

Although I learned a tremendous amount about myself, it was not until I came to the United States of America in 1988 that I realized some of my bad habits had to change before it was too late.

After signing up with Camp America in June of 1988, I arrived via bus from New York City to Hancock, New York. I was quickly introduced to a rough-looking fella named Jimmy, who gave me a couple of basic rules to live by: "You don't know shit from Shinola," and "You do as I say, not as I do." I had just learned my first two lessons in directive leadership.

I remember it well: I threw my smokes in the garbage with the intention of never smoking again. Not long after I arrived in camp, I walked into heaven when I entered the assigned house for my summer job: beer cans everywhere and heavy smoke lingering...with some funny smell mixed in. So much for leaving all my bad habits behind when I got off the bus in Hancock!

Just a couple of weeks later, I met a girl named Catherine in the OK Saloon, at which time my fate was sealed. Even though I didn't marry her, it did lead me to stay for much longer than my visa allowed. Not long after my first "Dear John" letter, I found myself all alone, searching for love and a green card.

In 1989, I married my first wife, Janice, who gave me three bundles of joy: Abigail, Kimberlie, and Erik. After getting our growing family settled, I owned a small bakery, deli, and pizzeria called Big Daddy; however, my itch for health care remained strong. Over the next few years, I earned my certifications as an emergency medical technician, a paramedic, and ultimately a flight paramedic.

Wherever I worked, I pursued positions of leadership. I took great joy in practicing my technical skills and finding opportunities to make process improvements. As a young leader, I grew a deep appreciation for individuals and their behaviors under different circumstances. My jobs during this time provided ample opportunity to coach and mentor for success.

I remember September 11, 2001, like it was yesterday: I made that dreadful call home, leaving a brief voice mail to say good-bye, not knowing what my day as a paramedic would hold in store.

Unlike many of our associates, I made it home that day; however, it left me thinking about my future and my desire for positivity and happiness. It was not long thereafter that Janice and I called it quits, allowing each of us to pursue happiness. We clearly had failed each other in more ways than one, but I have no regrets, as our marriage taught me valuable lessons about mistakes I promised myself I'd never repeat again.

In 2005, I sat on the couch at Rockland Paramedic Services Station 3, chatting with my paramedic partner, Bernadette, and wondering what we were going to do now that our first gray hairs had started to appear. I finally put pen to paper and developed my very first action plan, including realistic three- to five-year goals to earn my bachelor and master's degrees in business. I stuck to my plan and completed it on time—and only slightly over budget.

Toolbox

One-Year Plan	Three-Year Plan	Five-Year Plan
Goal	Goal	Goal
Action Plan	Action Plan	Action Plan

Make sure your goals meet the threshold of being "Specific, Measurable, Attainable, Realistic, and Timely."

In 2005, at Mama's Fish House in Maui, I married a second time, to Erica, the best nurse ever (I'm not biased, of course). Over the next four years, we welcomed our daughter, Maia, and son, Max, into our family.

Nothing gives me greater joy than watching my children grow into their own. Each of my special bundles of joy is unique in his or her own right, with dreams of exploring the world and making a difference. A parent couldn't wish for anything more.

By 2011, I was the proud owner of a BS, an MBA, a real-estate license, a pilot's license, and certification as a black-belt Six Sigma and LEAN provider. Determination and sticking to my SMART goals—plus lots of support from my family along the way—allowed me to realize my educational goals.

Now that you know a little more about me and my background, let's get back to the reason for this book. Over the years, I have developed a strong liking of process improvement and organizational development. I've had the opportunity to learn many different techniques, strategies, and philosophies from across different industries, including manufacturing and health care. Through observation of individuals and teams, I've realized that the magic in performance is less about staff's technical abilities and more about the individual's or teams behavioral capacity to change. In my experience, teams that embraced change came out on top at the end of the day more often than not.

Each successful team had one thing in common: it was led by a passionate and collaborative *positude* leader. It is the leader who sets the stage, who communicates a clear vision, who delivers with consistent passion, and who leads with humility. Teams with these secret ingredients consistently stood out for performance and satisfaction.

The challenge we face as leaders is the fact that we consistently promote our very best technical staff without proper support systems, mentorship, and coaching for success. After recognizing this gap, I felt the need to develop a countermeasure, from which the idea for a book was born.

I'm targeting our transitioning technical staff, such as doctors, nurses, technicians, and clerks, who are at risk of failure if we don't support them properly. If for nobody else, this book is dedicated as a countermeasure to the "Peter Principle," in support of our middle managers. As leaders, we need to recognize that we don't spend enough time developing this group, although we depend on them for just about everything we need.

It is my hope that you will learn from my experiences and choose a path that fits your needs to bring out the very best you have to offer. Life is a journey with lots of ups and downs; however, it is what we do with our downs that will determine how successful we will be.

As we transition to our strategies, skills, and experiences section of this book, make sure you adopt a *positive attitude*, or *positude*, before proceeding. Open your shoulders, sit up straight, take some deep breaths in just as you would to smell some beautiful roses, and exhale the way you would to blow out a candle. Clear your mind; be teachable; relate, don't compare; be open to new suggestions; and internalize the materials, even if you need to read them a few times. Only then will you get the most out of my writing.

Positude leadership is about a journey that starts on the next page, a personal journey full of learning, coaching, mentoring, sharing, growing, leading, inspiring, and teaching that will lead to success.

Throughout the text, you will find toolboxes with basic examples of ways to evaluate, assess, and develop your abilities to grow and lead. One such tool-kit item can be found on the next page; getting to know yourself and those you lead will make you that much more effective as a leader.

Invest in your team; invest in yourself.

Toolbox

As a leader, one needs to assess how well each team member is performing and identify opportunities to strengthen behavioral capacity, which is a strong predictor of performance.

If your budget allows, I would recommend you use a professional service to conduct an axiology exam or a PPI exam, otherwise Google *axiology*, and you will have a plethora of choices.

For those with a limited budget, I have provided below an example of how you can conduct your own basic personality and behavioral assessment. I strongly encourage you to have a clear understanding of the differences among IQ, EQ, and PQ before you get started.

$$\text{Performance} = (\text{Technical Abilities})(\text{EQ} \times \text{PQ})$$

Rate staff-member technical abilities   1   2   3   4   5

Rate staff-member emotional intel*   1   2   3   4   5

Rate staff-member positivity intel*   1   2   3   4   5

*Online you can find multiple free EQ/PQ assessment tools to get a more accurate score.

The total score provides a performance predictor. Use a dot plot to see how your team ranks in comparison to both each other and an established database. I suspect you will see a typical bell curve of low, middle, and high performers.

Chapter 1

Creating Your Own Mini Culture

Are you ready to be awesome? Are you ready to take charge of your own mini culture, or are you sitting back waiting to be bitten by the corporate-culture bug?

Cambridge Dictionary defines *culture* as "the way of life, especially the general customs and beliefs, of a particular group of people at a particular time."

Too many of us don't really understand what a culture is. I'm sure you have heard someone say, "Culture eats strategy for breakfast." But what does this actually mean? Can you *see* culture or *eat* strategy? No. However, you can certainly *feel* when you are in a bad culture or when management is executing an even worse strategy.

It's really no different from Step One of the Twelve Steps created by Alcoholics Anonymous, where one needs to admit to having a problem and acknowledge that life has become unmanageable. That's where most of the problems start: denial or just simple ignorance of the fact.

Let's make a deal: no matter where you work or what you do, we should agree that improvements can be made in both culture and strategy. Now that we have settled this important factor, let us start with exploring opportunities to improve both, at least on a personal level.

For starters, we need to identify vital components of culture before we start making improvements or investing more time in less relevant areas of operations.

Next, we will break each must-change area of operations down in greater detail from a thirty-thousand-foot level. Each of these areas will vary in each hospital or business; therefore, you will need to do some homework for your specific area of operations.

Toolbox

To be a successful *positude* leader, you need to have a visual reminder on your desktop of what must change. Copy and paste this to a place you will see daily.

Key components of what must change to produce an improved outcome:

- Manage performance and accountability
- Strengthen relationships
    - People skills
    - Emotional maturity
    - Train to higher capability
- Improve patient experience
- Improve support services
    - Information technology
    - Better financial information
- Change the culture
    - Commitment and ownership
    - Recognize good performance

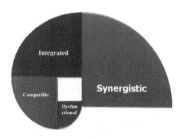

Performance Management and Accountability

Depending on what type of organization you work for, you may or may not have access to actual performance measures for your specific work units. Clinical performance measures are available in near real time; however, financial or efficiency performance metrics are not only difficult to obtain, but they are often reported months after the fact. As a manager, you will be held accountable as you will be holding your staff accountable...but how is this possible if you don't have performance measures to manage? If you were to visit a for-profit center, you would see performance measures at every turn, and it is a priority topic of conversation at every meeting; however, that represents less than 20 percent of all hospitals in the United States.

Instead of depending on others, as a manager, you need to make it a top priority to identify performance measures that need to be managed regularly.

A good place to start is a conversation with your boss, in which you ask for clarification on your supervisors expectations and discuss what performance measures are available to you, as well as what realistic outcomes he or she desires from the team. Before people can perform, they need to understand what is expected of them and how it is measured. This is true for any employee, from a frontline staff member all the way to an executive in the boardroom.

However, performance management and accountability are a whole lot more than just a metric goal you need to meet or exceed. Not to oversimplify performance management and accountability, but one should follow some basic rules of engagement:

1. Right people, right roles
2. Unified vision
3. Meaningful metrics
4. Accountability to self and team
5. Countermeasures to nonperformance

I'm not going to leave you to figure these steps out on your own; let me steer you in the right direction. Getting great at implementing these rules of engagement will take lots of practice and learning from inevitable failures along the way.

Right People, Right Roles

Jim Collins's *Good to Great* is worth reading on this principle.

All too often, we hire the best person for the job but not the *right* person for the job. Think back to your last hire; you posted a position, interviewed the five most qualified candidates who applied, and hired the best of the five available. The question is, did you hire the *right* person or just the best of the five available? Don't answer, because I already know what you'll say. We do this all the time. Jim Collins is very clear: don't settle on what is available; keep looking for the *right* person to improve your chances of long-term success. Your takeaway message is this: don't settle—find the *right* people for the *right* roles.

To improve your chances of performance management, it is an absolute must to develop a unified vision among your team members. Step into a conference room, close the door, and start your discussion with focus on your mission and desired outcomes. Before you get started, ask a question of each person in the room: Do we have a strong mutual respect among teammates? Do we have a common understanding and knowledge of our desired state? Are we in the right frame of mind to compromise and learn from one another? If even one of your teammates fails any of these basic questions, you have some work to do. Mutual respect and openness to learning are paramount to successful teams.

Do you have the *right* person in the *right* role? It's time to make some decisions, and it may be time to have some tough-love conversations with your team members. This is not easy, but it is absolutely necessary. Jump ahead for a few minutes and read some of my stories on this very topic to hone your skills in giving and receiving feedback.

Toolbox

Interviewing and selecting the right candidate:

1. Rate passion   1   2   3   4   5
2. Rate knowledge   1   2   3   4   5
3. Rate skill (tested by you)   1   2   3   4   5
4. Rate abilities   1   2   3   4   5

If a candidate does not score higher than sixteen points, you should continue to look.

Developing your team's unified vision:

1. Write down ten desirable team attributes.
2. As a team, decide on the top five attributes from question 1.
3. Question whether these attributes are aligned with your hospital's vision. Make adjustments as necessary.
4. Keep the team's vision statement under two hundred words.
5. Use creative writing to design three different versions of your team's vision statement.
6. Survey team at large, requesting feedback.
7. Incorporate feedback into final version.
8. Post in department for open-comment period.
9. Adjust as necessary.
10. Finalize, communicate, and market your team's new vision statement.

Now that the team has a unified vision, it's time to develop **S**pecific, **M**easurable, **A**ttainable, **R**ealistic, and **T**imely metrics that will provide near real-time feedback on performance. Make sure you have a good understanding of the difference between an outcome metric and a driver metric. For example, an outcome metric is your actual weight; a driver metric is a measure of the calories you consume each day, which affect the outcome metric. Invest enough time in this area to ensure you are targeting the right areas of operations and heading in the right direction. Measuring too late in the process can lead to great disappointment when it's time to present to your bosses or collect your bonuses.

None of this is relevant if you have a culture of unaccountability. Actually, I would argue that *accountability* is one of the nine dirty words not allowed to be said on public television. Do you work in a truly accountable organization? At best, maybe parts of your organization are, but this concept is a real struggle for all humankind. Why is it so difficult to create accountability among team members?

The answer is surprisingly simple: we are allergic to giving negative feedback to others and to setting performance expectations that will require an action if nonperformance continues to exist.

Some of you will disagree with me, but you are in the far minority and often are outcasts in your own work groups. I have seen all too often situations in which one manager holds folks accountable, while a manager of a different discipline working in the same unit does not. It spells conflict. Therefore, our conversation earlier about the need for a unified vision is crucial, and it should include equal accountability across all disciplines. There's no easy answer to this persistent phenomenon, and it will take discipline and teamwork to overcome this undesired side effect of being a performing manager.

To be accountable, one needs to *start* with self-accountability. Are you modeling the desired behavior? Are you holding your staff accountable? Are you providing feedback? Spend lots of time doing the right things right. As a leader, you never want to be accused of double standards or favoritism. Reassess your own performance on a regular basis, in part by conducting 360 reviews with some of your peers, supervisors, and staff members. It's a powerful tool to keep yourself honest and on track to being accountable and a high performer.

Equally important, your personal culture, as well as that of the organization, must include vigilance on team accountability without being overly harsh. Remember, we are trying to establish a culture of *positude*, collaboration, humility, and shared governance.

Holding people accountable starts with a crystal-clear vision and measures that show performance with great reliability. As a leader, you should adopt a five-level accountability system by escalating your expectation through asking, requesting, telling, directing, and then taking a trip to human resources for disciplinary resolution. As you practice this approach, you will see that you can be highly successful with most team members before you get to the final step.

Practice makes perfect; however, under performing measures will require a countermeasure when desired results are not achieved. As Einstein is believed to have said, the definition of insanity is completing the same actions over and over and expecting a different outcome.

Taking countermeasures is a team responsibility when nonperforming measures or team members fail to deliver or perform. Countermeasures can take the shape of anything from small adjustments to a complete overhaul or even abandonment of nonperforming projects or processes. They should be a topic of discussion at the end of every operations meeting: What do we need to change to get closer to the desired outcome?

Toolbox

Conducting 360 Performance Review

1. Select two staff members above, lateral, and below your position.
2. Request time on their calendars to conduct an in-person 360 review.
3. E-mail assessment forms to participants to allow time for preparation.
4. Be on time and prepared to listen twice as much as you talk.

Topic	Current Behavior	Future Behavior
What do I do well?		
What do I need to improve?		
What opportunities should I explore?		

Summarize your results from all participants, looking for trends, predictors, and opportunities for improvement. Use this tool to strengthen your *positude* leadership abilities.

Strengthen Relationships

In your personal pursuit to building a mini culture of excellence or as an organization in pursuit of performance management, it is vital to spend real time developing relationships not only with your peers but also with cross-departmental leaders and supporting disciplines. You may not need to be chummy with all of them, but you do need to understand the level of relationship needed to optimize performance. In some of my stories, I have outlined actual examples of how to build relationships and what types of relationships you need to have with close partners, including relationships that need to be abandoned immediately. At a minimum, you need to maintain functional relationships with coworkers not directly linked to your performance measures; meanwhile, you need to build synergistic relationships with ones on whom you depend for success.

Toolbox

Relationship Assessment

Go to page 155.

Improve Patient Experience

This should be the easiest of the topics to be considered, right? If patient or customer experience is *not* your top priority, press the red button now and delete this book. I will assume going forward that you are on the positive side or above the line in relation to the importance of patient experience.

In your team conversation about unifying your vision, patient experience, safety, and quality need to be cornerstones of the new house you are building.

Improving Support Services

My boss once said there are two types of folks in hospitals: those who take care of patients and those who take care of people who take care of patients. Undoubtedly, you belong to one of these groups and need support from administration, environmental services, information technology, building services, and the like.

The number-*one* complaint from providers on all levels is that they don't get to work at or above their licenses and frequently spend too much time getting access to systems that should be supported by the second group.

To build a new culture, don't forget to include support services in your relationship-building exercises or to bring them into your performance-management team. If you are a leader in support services, don't forget your role and mission to provide a service to those who provide patient care. Your mini culture should be based on service excellence, responsiveness, and timely delivery of services. Communications and transparency will greatly assist you with maintaining optimized relationships with your partners. All too frequently, individual partners don't understand the bigger picture and will become resentful toward their partners in support services. This can be prevented by taking the time to communicate, setting reasonable expectations, and following up until the request is completed.

I recommend you read *Change the Culture, Change the Game* by Roger Connors, as he does a really good job of taking readers on a journey of change. We previously agreed that you are not satisfied with your current state of affairs; something needs to change for you to get a different outcome. The foundation of your current personal culture is based on beliefs and experiences that you formed over a lifetime. Due to these experiences and beliefs, you take certain actions that deliver your current results. To change the outcomes, one needs to change one's actions.

Although it sounds simple and straightforward, it will be very difficult to make changes that will deliver your desired results unless you are willing to be teachable, open-minded, and ready to make *real* change. This is no different from when you start constructing your own new mini culture or that of your organization. Surround yourself with go-to people; build a strong, unified vision and even stronger partnerships; and take actions that are proven to be successful.

Change Model:

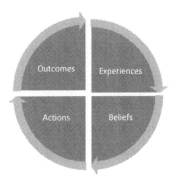

A lifetime of personal experiences installs long-term beliefs that will lead to actions aligned with your beliefs and past experiences.

Your actions will deliver your results. If you are not happy with your results, you need to change your perspectives and actions to realize a different outcome.

Having Fun

The fun portion of your new culture should be focused on rewards and recognition. Your cultural transformation is not complete unless you have set in stone commitments to celebrate success across the organization, starting within your own work unit and spreading to include all disciplines.

I can't say with enough passion that culture starts from the heart; it's not something that can be imposed upon you from headquarters or the C-suite. You have to believe in the change and feel commitment to providing excellence in every aspect of the business cycle, with your patients in the center of all your actions. You need to be committed, not just engaged in the culture change you want to see. Your energy and passion will rub off on the next employee, and if enough of you join the journey, it will affect the entire staff and institution before you know it. It has to start somewhere, so it might as well start with you. Be awesome!

If you change people's beliefs about how they should do their daily work and help them adopt the new beliefs you want them to hold, you will produce the actions you want them to take.
    —Unknown author

Toolbox

Performance-Management Work Sheet

Leadership Council Discussion

1. Why is performance management one of the top five issues that must change?
2. What is performance management? Define it.
3. What is currently being done with regard to performance management?
    a. What is working?
    b. What is not working?
4. What is acceptable performance management in the H and H culture? What is not?
5. Define the optimal performance-management process we want to follow at our hospital or business.

True Principles of Performance Management

1. Begin with desired outcomes in mind (expectations in terms of desired results and self-directed people).
2. Separate worth from performance.
3. Understand your staff perspectives—don't be judge, jury, and executioner.
4. Transfer ownership so people become self-directed.
5. Ensure accountability—no passes.
    a. Praise abundantly; recognize intrinsically.
    b. Provide honest, corrective feedback; be transparent without a hidden agenda; and build trust.
6. Focus on development and progress, not perfection.
7. Use a ratio of 3 positive to 1 negative comment to ensure a flourishing environment.

How to Do Performance Management

1. Clarify expectations in terms of desired results.
    a. Position profiles for physicians, nurses, PCAs, and clerks
    b. Expectations agreement
    c. Transfer ownership model

2. Focused feedback—tell them up front that you are going to let them know how they are doing.
    a. Use *appreciative focused feedback* that reinforces good performance
        i. Tell people what they did right; be specific and immediate.
        ii. Tell people how good you feel about what they did right and how it helps the organization and the other people who work here.
    b. Give *constructive, focused feedback* that offers positive and candid corrective suggestions.
        i. Tell people what they did wrong; be specific and immediate.
        ii. Tell people how you feel about what they did wrong.
        iii. Remind them how much you value them. Reaffirm that you think well of them but not of their performance in that particular situation.
        iv. Realize that when the correction is over, it's over.

Chapter 2

Four Strategies

Be Responsible—Love Those You Lead

This is one of my favorite topics, which is overlooked by too many leaders today. They undervalue and underestimate the power of a little *love* in the workplace. No, I'm not talking about the cuddly love that gets one in hot water with HR; I'm talking about genuinely caring for those who work with you and for you on all levels of the organization.

All too often, we get too absorbed in our own nonsense and have little capacity to be empathetic to anybody else. Check it out next time you walk into your building; observe where people's eyes are focused. You will see I'm right—they are staring at the floor with, at best, very little eye contact. We are in our own little worlds. Try something different tomorrow morning: as you enter the building, say simply but forcefully enough to be heard, "Good morning. How are you today?" or for departing staff after a long night, "Good morning. I hope you get some well-deserved rest today."

You will immediately see the difference in most people. They will pick up their heads, sort of make eye contact, and smile, at which time, unbeknownst to the smilers, a chemical is released in their brains that will make them feel happier. Don't stop with just the folks you see coming in; continue providing some love at every opportunity, and before you know it, you will see a return on your investment. It's just another integral part of building your personal mini-culture of excellence.

This is a small example of how you can make a difference every day; let's dig a little deeper to learn more about other opportunities to spread some love.

We will explore four strategies for creating a successful environment:

1. Love those you lead.
2. Lead through context.
3. Ensure a successful environment.
4. Use the power of focus.

Love Those You Lead

It is your responsibility as a leader to create a caring environment and get to know your staff on a personal level. It does not mean you need to go to dinner on Friday night or be expected to go to every communion, bar mitzvah, or wedding, but it does mean you need to show interest in personal-interest stories. You need to make time for your staff not only from a perspective of accountability but with empathy and caring for the person you encounter, taking some time to listen without always resolving problems.

A strategy I adopted some time ago to ensure I have time on the calendar to round with staff is to schedule some fake meetings—just make sure I follow through and get away from my office and computer.

Soon you will be receiving as much love as you will be giving. Frontline staff, especially, has a need to be heard and acknowledged; there's no better way of doing that than with some face time. Learn to enjoy this time with your staff; it will pay off tenfold.

Lead through Context

One of the most important messages you can ever deliver to your staff is one that has real context that is relatable, understandable, and translatable. All too often, leaders say a lot without saying the right things; more is not always better. As a leader, you have to really think through the message you are about to deliver. Who is your audience, what is it you are trying to say, can staff relate to it, and does it come from the heart? On some occasions, you are better off going the extra mile and explaining it in language your audience understands, especially the "why" of your request for performance or change. If your staff understands the why, they can attach emotion to the cause, get skin in the game, and see a finish line in the distance. It's only natural to want to win as long as you know what winning looks like.

Ensure a Successful Environment

Sitting in an old chair behind a rickety desk with a carpet smelling of mildew is not going to make you feel like a winner, nor will it make you feel good about yourself, your unit, or the work you perform. You cannot underestimate the power of a successful environment, and it doesn't stop in the office itself. Everything you see and everywhere you go can influence how you present yourself, think, or act. As a leader, you have to develop great situational awareness to identify such areas and rectify them in short order. On occasion, and especially in environments where money is short, you can come together and make it work. Dress for success; set your office up to facilitate learning, coaching, and mentoring—clutter free, of course.

Next, it is time to clear your brain; no more rent-free living for those who have occupied that space for too long. You need to be fresh and open; you have to able to make decisions with clarity. This is going to take some practice on your part, but it's a worthwhile exercise. Last, staff members need a space where they feel safe, which is unlikely to be in your office. Create fear-free spaces throughout your work unit where you can visit staff in their natural environment.

Use the Power of Focus

A very wise man once told me that more is not always better. Too many of us take on responsibilities beyond our abilities of effectiveness simply due to an inability to say no. Are we making the right decision for us and our patients, clients, and coworkers? Probably not. We lose effectiveness and frequently end up failing when overextended. There's actually some truth to the fact that five or more projects at one time will lead to failure, while three to five projects at one time will deliver partial results with poor sustainability; however, focused attention on one or two projects at one time optimizes both outcomes and long-term success. This doesn't mean you should stop paying your bills, go home at 2:00 p.m., or no longer worry about the future; what it means is that the power of focus will allow you to be successful far more often. The power of focus is not only limited to working on only one or two projects; also focus your project's scope to something that is attainable.

It's now time to take it from a thirty-thousand-foot level down to ground level using four strategies to building lasting and loving relationships with your staff and coworkers.

1. Know them.
2. Understand their perspectives.
3. Show tough love.
4. Identify intrinsic drivers.

Know Them

How well do you really know your staff and coworkers? Can you tell me a story about each of your staff members? What makes them engaged in the workplace? There are many questions, and most of us know little about the folks who work with and for us. Are we really too self-absorbed to care, or do we just not make the time to get to know a bit more about the people with whom we spend more time than we do with our own significant others?

I'm not advocating that you need to go to happy hour or invite any of them to your house for dinner; however, building a strong partnership requires you to get to know the person beyond a first and last name.

Many years ago, I started asking a standard question at the end of every meeting; I asked my staff members to share a significant moment in their lives with the team—for example, birthdays, weddings, or graduations. Once staff members feel comfortable, you will hear amazing stories. Each of these stories will allow you to get to know this person a bit more, but more importantly, you have an opportunity to relate and build a genuine relationship going forward.

You can't invest enough time in this strategy; it will pay off in many ways.

Understand Their Perspectives

How is this strategy any different from the one we just addressed? Getting to know someone on a more personal level will provide you valuable insights and allow you to shape a new relationship going forward.

Understanding their perspectives should be explored in different ways, including walking a mile in their shoes. It's the most powerful way to appreciate one another's pain. For example, imagine you have a high-performing staff member show up late every morning to the point that you can't ignore it any longer. Traditionally, we would have disciplined this staffer and moved on to the next task, leaving this staff member in despair. A *positude* leader, however, would take the time to find out *why* the staff member comes in late each shift and would work together with him or her to resolve this issue to both sides' satisfaction, creating a win-win scenario. Another example would be to sit in a busy practice and look through the lens of a provider to see what could be done by someone on a lower level. A short walk in someone's shoes can provide a perspective that otherwise goes unnoticed.

Show Tough Love

Utopia in health care would be perfection at every turn, which is unlikely to happen, but something we *can* commit to is taking 100 percent responsibility without making excuses for the actions we take. We fail at this more often than anything else. We just love to place blame with others; point the finger at them; or provide a barrage of excuses for why something happened, with little or no self-reflection.

Only very emotionally mature members of the organization will elevate themselves and give a sincere apology when necessary or, at minimum, will feel equally responsible for a poor outcome, regardless of who is to blame.

As an individual within an organization of many, one must see oneself as part of a team, where responsibility is shared and successes are celebrated together. With the best teams in history—particularly in the game of soccer, where every player has a distinctive role to play—the team wins or loses together, with the players feeling equally responsible for the outcome. It really is the difference between a *team* of players and a *group* of players. A *team* is bonded and invested emotionally in the action and outcome, while a *group* will place blame on those who failed the team.

We need to show love throughout the organization and work relentlessly to become high-performance teams. Love will bring people together, but it won't necessary solve tough problems. Tough love is still very much part of a *positude* leader's repertoire. It is essentially important to coach, mentor, or even discipline team members if necessary, using your very best vital-conversation skills.

As a leader, take a few steps back and observe your team with an open mind to assess whether you are managing a *group* or a *team*. Are your team members emotionally mature enough to take responsibility for a failure, no matter who failed on the team? Most *teams*, and certainly not *groups*, are not ready for the 100/0 culture (100 percent shared responsibility/zero excuses), and you will have your work cut out for you. Utilizing the strategies and skills outlined in both chapters and stories will provide you the guidance to attain a 100/0 culture of excellence. Your players are ready to play; some need a little love, and others a little tough love, to get heading in the right direction.

Leading by example is never more important than in a 100/0 environment. You will slip and go back to an old habit of blaming, but it is what you do after you realize you have slipped that is the most important thing as a responsible leader; you apologize for slipping up, take responsibility, and learn from your experiences.

Identify Intrinsic Drivers

Throughout all the chapters and stories, I consistently outline the importance of needing to manage the individual, not just the team. Each person in the organization comes from his or her own background, with deeply personalized beliefs and experiences that result in actions that deliver outcomes. If you were to hold everybody to a single standard, you would quickly lose the personality and creativity of your individual staff members. Therefore, it is critical that you look at each person as an individual who is driven by different beliefs, likes, and needs.

Don't believe me? Here's a simple little exercise: go to the nearest five staffers in your work area and ask them what their favorite animal is. It is highly unlikely that you will get the same answer, or even two of the same, in this small sample group. This is powerful evidence that we all are a bit different from one another and therefore should be managed based on individual intrinsic drivers to optimize outcomes and performance.

Take a quick look ahead at the toolbox on the next page, which contains fourteen different intrinsic drivers for engagement that you can use as a starting point of conversation as you meet with each person. As a leader, it is your responsibility to get the most out of each position and person; one way of doing this is to develop a relationship with your team members and identify their unique intrinsic drivers for engagement.

You will need to take the time to introduce this exercise properly and, more importantly, to use the information gleaned from each person.

Create a simple Excel spreadsheet, and refer to it at least monthly to ensure you have taken concrete steps toward feeding your team members' intrinsic drivers.

Ignore it, and you run the risk of being discredited as insincere by your staff members. Keep yourself honest by setting a reminder on your calendar to perform an intrinsic-driver checkup.

Toolbox

Individual Intrinsic-Driver Assessment Tool

1. Create a simple Word document on your letterhead.
2. Develop a power paragraph describing your desire to become a better leader with focus on each individual.
3. Ask each individual to carefully assess from the listings or to add any intrinsic values that would make him or her feel more engaged at work.
4. Introduce your request for information to each person face-to-face. This will show you are sincere, and it will allow time for clarification.
5. Request the return of your assessment tool within one week.
6. Catalog your results and refer to them frequently.
7. Make every attempt possible to minimally address one intrinsic driver per staff member on a weekly basis to optimize return on investment.

Intrinsic Drivers		
Need me	Resource me	Focus/direct me
Know/care about me	Empower me	Grow me
Inform me	Inspire me	Include me
Challenge me	Be abundant with me	Help me achieve
Hear me	Appreciate me	

Chapter 3

Five Essential Skills to *Positude* Leadership

Deep Listening

Are you really listening—receiving a message and processing it before carefully formulating a proper response, which, at times, could occur the next day rather than in the next minute?

By nature, we are not very skilled listeners, especially alpha men; we are problem solvers and have little empathy or time to really listen to what we are being told. (For the record, some women are equally guilty of this lack of caring.) Sometimes the speaker or person seeking help just wants to be heard or to be understood and validated; only then—if at all—will he or she be open to help.

The helper wants to solve the problem, fix the issue, make it all better, and get credit for being the hero who made everything better.

Do you see yourself in any of this? Most people can relate and therefore can become more intense listeners by exercising discipline in the way they ask questions, how they request clarification, and how they validate what they've heard by providing a synopsis of the helpee's statements. Only then can one assess when and what the appropriate response should be. Sometimes less is better, and the time to respond is not immediately; it may be best to let the situation sink in before responding—depending on the scenario, of course.

Listening is very difficult, and it will take some time to get very good at it. I still struggle at times, as I want to fix issues immediately but need to remind myself that, in some instances, it's more important for someone to be heard. Keep trying; get better with every conversation you have.

Apologize When Appropriate

The power of a sincere, well-timed apology should not be underestimated. It's a shame more of our leaders don't recognize the benefits of taking responsibility without making excuses and of delivering an apology from the heart.

We have all witnessed firsthand a time when something went wrong and finger-pointing started shortly thereafter. What a missed opportunity for a leader. It takes emotional maturity and understanding the human psychology to deliver, without hesitation, an empathetic apology from the heart.

Let's be crystal clear though: As a leader, you don't need to become an apology machine. Doing so will discredit you and will potentially bring down morale.

Be a *positude* leader who is emotionally mature, assesses each failure from multiple angles, and is prepared to shoulder the responsibility without placing blame on his or her staff members. A *positude* leader will see a failure as an opportunity to succeed and learn.

Feedback

The necessity of vital conversations when creating your mini culture of excellence is unquestionable. When was the last time you executed a flawless vital conversation? Most of you will be scratching your heads right now and, after some deep soul-searching, will conclude that you have avoided more vital conversations than you have ever conducted.

Highly effective leaders, and certainly *positude* leaders, will have learned to embrace vital conversation to strengthen a relationship, even when coaching, mentoring, or counseling an underperforming staff member.

I deeply appreciate the human psychology and fears in critically addressing a shortcoming, but failure to learn *how* to conduct a vital conversation will lead to stagnation in your career.

Gone are the days when you call someone into your office and go up one side and down the other to address failures in the workplace.

Great organizations will have a code of conduct, service-excellence, or workplace-violence policy that prohibits such behaviors. If your organization doesn't have this in place, start working on one.

Back to the vital conversation. It is inevitable that you will experience a moment or conduct that is less than desirable and in need of discussion. Instead of addressing this in front of others, start by creating a safe environment where a discussion can be held with the mind-set of creating a win-win outcome based on principles of mutual respect, common bond, and teachability.

After carefully selecting the right place to conduct such a conversation, start by using your deep-listening skills; give your staff member some time to explain him- or herself, ask appropriate questions to clarify the situation, and repeat a summary of what you were told to ensure you are on the same page. Take your time asking and answering questions; you *must* get this right.

Next, address the core issue directly and firmly but with respect, outlining a desired behavior under similar circumstances. By remaining open-minded and teachable yourself, you can start the process of healing and negotiating a win-win scenario.

Using the 80/20 rule, you will be able to create a win 80 percent of the time and see a changed behavior and improved engagement by the staff member. If it goes super well, your staff members will be able to reflect upon their own behaviors and show gratitude at some point in time for confronting the issue head-on.

Many of us become blind to our own bad behaviors, and a structured vital conversation can bring *positude* back into the workplace and significantly strengthen your relationships.

It's like exercising a muscle: if you don't do it often enough, you will never get great at it.

Developing a Common Bond

In which direction is the ship heading? If you get a different answer from each discipline, you can rest assured that there's no common bond on your interdisciplinary team. Sadly, this is an all-too-common phenomenon in health care. The likely root cause can be found in lack of understanding of each role in the overall picture. Leadership should take responsibility and work twice as hard to bring all disciplines to the table to develop strong interpersonal relationships based on a common understanding and bond.

As a leader, you have to pay particular attention to assuring all team players are singing from the same sheet of music and prefer using the same notes. It is important to start with clearly defining your objectives and carefully selecting key stakeholders from all disciplines to be represented on your team. Only then can you start with development of a common bond among all team members.

Don't cut corners, or it will bite you in the buttocks at a later time. Use your acquired strategy of leading through context to drive home the need for alignments and a strong bond between teammates.

Make It a Safe Place

This is the last of the major skills you need to develop as a *positude* leader. I cannot overstate the importance of getting this right more often than not. Everything you will do with your teams or individuals you manage is based on your ability to have great situational awareness and ensure that you choose the right environment for the actions you are undertaking.

A safe place is unlikely to be your office or even a conference room; a safe place is defined by the person you are meeting with, but it doesn't end with just picking the right location.

Being safe requires you, as the *positude* leader, to be aware of your body language, your tone of voice, your approach to a difficult conversation, or even the way you celebrate successes. If you think this is easy, think again. It's highly unlikely that you are paying much attention to this right now, simply because I didn't point it out to you, or, more likely, because nobody has had the courage to tell you what you need to hear.

The next time you need to do a performance evaluation, go to your staff members' offices instead of bringing them to you. Start the conversation on a personal note, recognize something positive that has taken place, and point out how they were a positive influence. Get into the flow of the conversation before transitioning into the meat-and-potatoes part of the evaluation. Use this skill when you have to bring bad news, introduce new mandates, or celebrate successes.

The last piece of the puzzle, which is extremely important—especially for us who tower over most people—is to sit down to reduce the height differential. Like it or not, one's height can be very intimidating to the opposing party, which will inhibit a fluent conversation with bilateral flow of information, thought, and challenges.

Be mindful of personal space; it differs from person to person. Violate this rule, and you will create an unsafe learning and development environment.

We have worked our way through five essential skills for a *positude* leader. What you should do next is reread these few pages and internalize what is suggested to you and ways to practice to build up stamina. Using these five essential skills will allow you to get to the next level of performance. *Change the culture, change the game* means changing your personal way of presenting yourself to drive toward a desired outcome. A bodybuilder doesn't become a muscleman overnight; it takes true dedication to the craft and an untold number of hours in the gym to get the desired results. To become a *positude* leader, it will take just as much dedication to transform your habits into your newly desired leadership style.

As you go forward, at each interaction, practice your newly acquired skills, and you will see that it becomes your natural behavior over time. Accept that we are humans and are not flawless; however, if you are truly mindful of your mindfulness, you will self-recognize missteps and correct them at your next opportunity.

Chapter 4

One Hundred Experiences

Up to this point, you should feel that you have gained knowledge and skills for becoming a highly effective *positude* leader. Over the next hundred pages, you will gain insight based on true stories and experiences that will bolster your abilities to lead through *positude*.

Relate; Don't Compare

Each experience will contain a problem statement, an example, and a solution based on personal experiences over the past twenty years.

I have unidentified all coworkers; however, I'm eternally grateful for their positive and negative experiences. They have given me the opportunity to grow as a professional and become a *positude* leader.

Open your mind, relax your brain, and go on a journey of learning, relating, and sharing.

Chapter 5

Is Your Team a Team?

It has been an exciting week in the sports world, to say the least. In the NBA finals, Cleveland became champs, and I'm watching the final match of the Copa America—Argentina versus Chile in overtime—as I'm writing this story! (Congrats, Chile!)

There's no question that we are seeing teams at work where collaboration rules the day. Can you say the same of *your* team?

Not too long ago, I got to observe a group of team members in a team-building session. I was under the impression that this group of staff members worked well together and looked after one another. Looks can be deceiving.

It didn't take more than five minutes, as they all sat in a circle, to observe that something was desperately wrong with this group. Their body language was screaming dysfunction, resentment, and discordance.

It was time for some honest critical feedback and a reset of the team dynamics. I stepped out at this point and let a very capable coach take over to start with the first step of recovery, by getting the team to admit they were merely a group of staffers working in the same area and not clicking on all cylinders.

I have never seen a *group* of people win much of anything; however, I can think of the Chicago Bulls, Utah Jazz, Warriors, and now Cleveland, who elevated a team of players into the stratosphere of performance. How did they do it?

They understood their mission and their individual roles; they put *team* before *self* or *ego*! The *team* came together and celebrated wins and mourned losses, spending numerous hours analyzing *why* they lost, without placing blame. The *team* looked at failure as an opportunity for improvement.

Your lesson: don't assume you have a team working for you. Take your time to observe them in a group session, ask the right questions in a safe environment, and take advantage of this to either start building a team or to strengthen your team.

Teams win; groups waste effort.

Chapter 6

Finding the Right Teammates

Four simple, powerful, and meaningful words to remember: passion, skill, knowledge, and ability.
Which one should be a given, one we should not compromise on?

Passion can't be taught; you either have it, or you don't. All of my go-to staff members have one thing in common: they are passionate about the work they do. Of course, possessing skill, knowledge, and ability only enhances the staff member to become a high-performing teammate. Skill, knowledge, and ability can be gained through coaching, mentoring, and repetition; however, *passion* is part of your DNA.

This is where our previously discussed concept of *right people, right job* comes into play. It's a great basic rule, but I would add one more requirement we should not compromise on: right passion for the right job! Passionate team members are most often go-to personalities—they are performers, they are teachable, they are loyal and caring, and they will go above and beyond. These types of staff members have the right balance of *positude* leadership.

Take your time selecting the *right* team members, because adding a "just OK" member to your team will only slow you down. You will have inherited lots of "just OK" team members who will need to be managed *up* or managed *out* of the organization. There are lots of useful tips to come in regard to developing, coaching, and mentoring staff members to get the most out of each individual.

Tell me about your passionate teammates.

Chapter 7

What Is Your Leadership Style?

My first reaction would be to say that different scenarios call for different leadership styles. My personal preference is being a servant and collaborative leader, which has been very successful for me over the years and uses escalation techniques whenever necessary.

What I mean by escalation is that we should always be centered, collaborative servants and lead with positive and passionate attitudes. Starting from this basis, we lead through context, provide clear expectations, and *ask* our teammates to meet those expectations within a set timeframe that varies from project to project depending on urgency and impact. By outlining your expectations, assessing the behavioral capacity of your teammates, and asking them to provide a solution and deliver the required results, you are, in essence, building a psychological contract with your team members, which will more likely lead to success, because they are empowered to come up with solutions.

To ensure success, we need to be accountable; therefore, we need to regularly check in on the contract status and progress made. If expectations are not met, we need to assess *why* before we escalate to *requesting*, then *telling*, and finally *directing* our team members and leaders.

Each step should be considered carefully and escalated on a predetermined timeline. Needless to say, if after *directing*, desired results are not delivered or actions are not taken, it is time for a performance-improvement plan to be enacted through HR; however, you'll see that most often you will get great cooperation and results simply by *asking*.

Being a servant collaborative leader, you will get the results you desire, elevate staff engagement to new levels, and celebrate successes.

What is your leadership style, and how is it working for you?

Chapter 8

Every Day Is a New Beginning

No matter what yesterday felt like, if you are lucky enough to rise in the morning, you have a new opportunity to love, learn, teach, share, mentor, and accomplish. Never take such opportunities for granted.

From failures, we grow stronger, and we will only fail if we refuse to learn and adjust from our failures.

Therefore, every day is a new beginning and, as a leader, another opportunity to serve, encourage, engage, and collaborate so we won't make the same mistakes again. Instead, you will prosper and provide excellence, no matter what position you are in.

I live by a simple rule: yesterday is a bad check, and tomorrow is not here, so I'd better pay attention and appreciate what I have today.

Be mindful of your mindfulness!

Chapter 9

Reluctance to Change

As human beings, we are forever changing, from the time we are born till the day we die. Many of us are highly resistant to this forever-changing process and do all kinds of silly things to prevent aging through exercise, surgery, diet, creams, pills, and so on. Why would we *not* be resistant to change in the workplace? It only makes sense.

The problem is that *change* is inevitable, and if we don't outpace the changes, we will be left behind. Simply look at the history of Blockbuster Video, a top-of-the-line company on the leading edge of technology when VHS and Betamax were still cool. They adapted when we changed technologies to CD and DVD; however, they quickly fell behind and didn't adapt to change in time to convert systems to streaming technology and the low-cost DVD kiosk at every supermarket in town. The result: out of business. The cause: reluctance to change.

So when one asks, "Why such reluctance to *change*?" the answer is simple: it's human nature for the vast majority of the population. Therefore, inspirational leadership is necessary to break through the reluctance.

We need to lead through *context* by answering *why* there's a need for change. We need to provide safety and security and lead on the path of change.

How do we best explain change or what it feels like? Try this simple exercise with your staff; ask them to write their full names with their dominant hands twenty times. Pause and ask them what it felt like. You know the answers: *comfortable, safe, normal, part of me*, and so on. Now ask them to do exactly the same with their nondominant hands and pause after every fifth time. You will get answers from *reluctant, uncomfortable, painful,* and *awkward* to "I'm getting used to it," and finally it will be the new norm if they don't have a choice to go back to the old way of doing things. It is an eye-opening exercise.

So reluctance to change is human nature; as long as we are sensitive to this and lead change to become the new norm in a safe environment, we can be more successful in staying ahead.

Be the change you desire.

Chapter 10

What to Do If Your Project Fails

Bury your head in the sand, blame everybody but yourself, tell everybody your project wasn't resourced right and they just don't get it—see a trend? It is *their* fault *your* project failed.

With a mind-set such as this one, you are doomed to repeat this pattern over and over until one day you wake up and accept responsibility for your failures.

Taking responsibility regardless of who is at fault makes you that much more effective as a leader, especially if you convert a failure into an opportunity to learn, study, adjust, and try again.

Leaders who never fail don't try hard enough. It's like running in place; you will never go anywhere.

So what should you do after a project fails? Take a deep breath, take a few steps backward, and when ready, start dissecting the reasons *why* your project failed. It's like a root-cause analysis, using the five whys to get to the bottom without placing blame. Only then can you start studying and learning from past missteps.

The most common reasons *why* projects fail are lack of communication to target audience, lack of common vision, failure to bring value, lack of project champions, lack of common understanding, not enough support for the project for long enough, poor project metrics, and the like.

The key takeaway messages are to take a calculated risk, not to be afraid to fail, convert failures into opportunities, and make sure you work from a solid foundation, including mutual respect, common understanding, common bond and vision, teachability, and the right people in the right roles. Along with meaningful measures, this will set you up for likely success.

I can, and I will...a little positude plus will goes a long way to reaching your destination.

Chapter 11

Gain Strength through Adversity

Have you ever been told no, been turned down for a job, been yelled at by your boss, or been caught up in a mess? I'm sure we have all been there at one time or another.

Sadly, many are discouraged by such events to the extent that they end up making life-altering decisions based on emotions rather than strength.

Losing at work, in a relationship, or just in life will jolt the best of us through the multiple stages of grief: denial, anger, bargaining, depression, and acceptance. Some of us go through the stages in minutes or hours; others will take days, weeks, or longer to recover.

Only after acceptance can you gain strength from adversity by understanding, learning, and adjusting, making sure appropriate course directions are made in a clear state of mind and not in a period of great confusion.

Being humble, taking responsibility, and making an apology will allow you to personally and professionally grow to another level.

Remember what I have said before: those who run in place and don't take risks will rarely face real adversity but will also not change or transform anything.

Go out on a limb, be brave, and go for it—believe in yourself and be confidently humble.

Chapter 12

Are You Ready for a 360?

Have you ever done a 360 review? Opening oneself up for critique with the expectation of improvement after shared goals have been set is kind of scary and not for the fainthearted.

If you have never done a 360 review, it is very simple: ask three folks above, below, and on the same peer level to spend fifteen to thirty minutes with you to outline your strengths and accomplishments, your weaknesses, and your opportunities. To get the best results, e-mail or call them a few days ahead of time to discuss expectations, allowing some time to prepare and make it truly meaningful.

After you get your results back, categorize them by level of review and look for trends between surveys. I'm sure you will find commonalities, which will allow you to focus on the most significant opportunities for improvements.

The power of feedback can't be overstated. Be brave, take a chance, and include someone who might not be your greatest cheerleader.

There's more to come on what to do with information gleaned from your 360.

A proper 360 is a window to your future.

Chapter 13

Man Down

We have all been there so many times: finally hitting a stride and getting performance from your team before the rug is pulled from underneath you due to a vital resignation, sick calls, FMLAs, or, worse, involuntary downsizing.

Frequently, you will see teams fall apart if a key stakeholder goes missing. Why is that?

The most common reason is due to the fact that teams and processes become specific-person dependent without redundancy or diversity. Stop what you are doing and think for just a second: *Do I have a team or process built around a specific leader or staff member?*

We all do and need to build in redundancy and succession plans in case of a loss to ensure processes can function equally well 24/7/365.

It's also a great opportunity to develop your teammates and leaders alike. One of the most important contributions a leader can make is to ensure systems are clicking regardless of who came to work that day.

Great teams always step up to the plate and cover the gaps; if one discipline is down a leader, it's time to lend a hand and fill the gap, not point out their weaknesses.

More importantly, working together is like a team sport: some of us play defense, and others play offense; however, when the team wins or loses, we should celebrate or reflect together—it's a *we* environment, not an *I* environment.

Great teams continue to function even when they are a man down.

Chapter 14

New Minute Manager, a Quick, Powerful Read

Very few of us love to read or even like to read; however, most effective staff members, managers, and leaders will make time to read.

You should make it a point to add calendar slots to your daily schedule to read for fifteen to thirty minutes to keep up with the forever-changing world around you.

A good place to start is *One-Minute Manager*, which authors Ken Blanchard, PhD, and Spencer Johnson, MD, have updated to include some additions with an emphasis on sharing.

Once you get settled in, it will take no more than ninety minutes to consume every last page with a thirst for more. However, it's certainly written with our attention spans in mind. After you go through the book once, you should sleep on it and read it one more time to ensure the finer points have sunken in. Only practice makes perfect.

More is not always better. A valuable lesson within these pages speaks simply to focused goals, creating wins, praise, and redirection through real-time feedback, all the while letting staff members know how valuable they really are.

It sounds so simple, and it actually is; we just have a hard time letting go and trusting others.

One-Minute Manager *is a powerful lunchtime read for champions.*

Chapter 15
Why Goal Setting Is Essential to Success

Have you ever had a boss who wanted you to be great, do great things, be a winner, succeed, perform, and bring home the bacon but who failed to define what great looked like and didn't set goals or targets? We have all been there at one time or another.

It's like playing darts at 3:00 a.m. with the lights off. You go for the bull's-eye, but you don't even know where the dartboard is hung. How frustrating is that? Who is to blame, you or your boss? Your boss took for granted that you knew what he or she was aiming for, but you failed to ask the right questions to define his or her expectations.

No matter what, performance should be based on measurable metrics and realistic goals. Personally, I prefer using *SMART* goals for each of our improvement projects and performance goals: **S**pecific, **M**easurable, **A**ttainable, **R**ealistic, and **T**imely.

Most importantly, we need to agree on *what* we are measuring, *how* we are measuring, and *when* we are measuring to ensure consistency and accountability. I also prefer realistic *step goals* instead of just a target to aim for. We need to celebrate wins along the way to keep our staff members excited. Ones who receive rewards along the way likely will be more productive, and rewards can be as simple as a personal acknowledgment in the form of a thank-you note, gift card, or pizza party for the team.

Turn on the lights, tell me your expectations, guide me in the right direction, and support me along the way, and I will give you my absolute best to meet your goals and expectations.

Be SMART; keep it real.

Chapter 16

Do You Praise Enough?

Can you remember the last time you received a compliment at work? I'm almost 100 percent sure you do and still talk about it with your peers or proudly display your *thank-you* note somewhere in your workplace. It's only human nature that we like to receive affirmation for the things we do every day.

Let's turn it around: When was the last time you took a few minutes to handwrite a thank-you card to someone who made your day better or went above and beyond?

Nearly 80 percent of you will answer that with a blank stare. We tend to provide more negative feedback than we take the time to praise someone. This is a bad habit we need to break if we really want to unlock the magic in our staff members.

Get to know your staff members, know what drives them to be successful, and know their intrinsic values and how to engage them.

Set realistic goals and give praise when goals are met or real effort is made toward meeting goals. Your staff members will respond in kind, just as you do when your boss takes the time to give you praise.

The value of a compliment is priceless.

Chapter 17

How to Best Provide Redirection

I'm not sure what is worse: getting negative feedback on something I did three months ago or being called to my supervisor's office for an unknown reason. Both circumstances can cause unnecessary frustration and anxiety.

Let's assume you started with crystal-clear goals and expectations a few weeks or months ago but have failed to deliver the desired results. You are not happy and are getting pressure from your superiors to get the job done. What should you do next? Go fix it yourself or have that difficult conversation? Why do we tend to avoid difficult conversations? Nearly 100 percent of the time, when we give constructive and timely feedback, staff members are responsive and appreciate honesty, clarity, and timeliness in a safe setting. Avoidance or waiting too long to provide feedback will have a directly inverse effect, leading to frustration and underperformance by all involved.

Here's my recommendation for providing a redirect: meet in a safe environment to provide feedback (not your office), provide feedback in near real time, review project goals to ensure alignment, review performance metrics, suggest corrective action to meet expectations, and agree to meet again. Show appreciation to your staff member.

Getting and giving feedback is essential to your long-term success; one just needs to make sure it's done in an environment conducive to learning.

Chapter 18

Why Don't We Share Our Best Practices?

The question really should be, "Why do we feel the need to reinvent the wheel?" Do you think working in a vacuum delivers better results? Why is it that we are so very protective of our own processes—especially those that work well?

I can understand not sharing with your direct competitors, but within the same corporation or even the same work unit, there should be zero reasons not to share best practices.

I think our need to win or outperform others gets in the way of delivering service excellence, being highly efficient, bringing cost savings, or increasing revenue. Some would rather *win* than share; however, we should all strive to be *winners*.

Collectively, we are stronger, better, leaner, and more efficient than any one of us is on our own.

It takes real leadership to empower and engage the staff to share best practices that will benefit the bottom line, especially your patients, clients, or even shareholders.

A simple approach would be to invite aligned work units to meet and report on progress they have made; organize a roundtable discussion or conference on a specific topic. Don't overcomplicate matters. If you organize it, they will come!

A little friendly competition will yield many great shared best practices.

Chapter 19

What to Do with Low Performers

Jack Welch once said that cutting the bottom 10 percent of your low-performing workforce would bring transformation and performance.

Some leaders hang onto this philosophy and would like to implement it in their own environments but often run into a brick wall (not built by Donald J. Trump), only to find it's not all that simple. Actually, it is often a very time-consuming and draining process, especially in a heavy union environment.

So what to do instead? Remember, my glass is always half-full; therefore, I prefer to spend some time with low performers to see *why* they are disengaged and what it would take to reengage them.

Being both a realist and a pragmatist, I'm not delusional in my thinking that everybody can be converted; I have found also that the vast majority can be made into contributing members of the workforce. Collectively, we need to be creative and mindful when exploring the options with low performers.

You should start by carefully listening to their stories. They each have one, and most are well aware of their lack of productivity or participation. Next, it's your turn; take the time to set the stage. Carefully outline *why* we need every staff member to be engaged, then express how it feels when they don't play nicely in the sandbox. Let this sink in a bit before transitioning to the negotiation phase of the meeting. By now, you have outlined the needs of the organization and can ask where the low performer can become an active and engaged employee who will be productive and goal oriented once again.

Applying the 80/20 rule, 80 percent of the low performers will express interest to be engaged in an area that connects with them emotionally, which is sometimes within their workplace or in another department. This is your opportunity to seal the deal, come to an agreement on how to proceed, set some realistic goals, and meet with them frequently until goals are met.

A word of advice: I have learned this the hard way myself—never promise something you can't deliver. Live by the rule *underpromise; overdeliver.*

Chapter 20

What Works Best? Asking versus Telling

Being told what to do is not very engaging to me. Do you agree? Most likely you do. It takes any sense of creativity and flexibility out of our ability to perform or produce.

There's a right time to be told. As effective leaders, we should not start by telling but rather should start by asking.

As leaders, on any level of the organization, we need to get things done, regardless of where you work or what you do. The old-fashioned way was either do it yourself or tell others to do it for you.

Which staff member is more productive, the one who is *told* what to do or the one who understands *why* it needs to be done? Simple answer, of course: staff members who understand *why* something needs to be done are more engaged and will be far more responsive once you *ask* them to do something.

As a *positude* leader, always start with leading through context and asking for staff participation by setting a clear vision and realistic goals. If staff is nonresponsive, then we can always resort to telling them what to do. You will see significant success with just asking, and it has a way of building respect and trust as well.

Ask, request, and tell before directing; it really works.

Chapter 21

How to Recruit for Success

This has to be one of the most difficult things we do. We post a position and select a bunch of résumés based upon some loose parameters before we invite the selected candidates in for an interview.

At last, we get to sit down with candidates who are nervous, shaky, and stressed to the point that they really are no longer the same people who applied for the job. Next, the crucial first impression and introductions. Love those soaking-wet handshakes, don't you? Over the next ten to fifteen minutes, you get to figure out if the candidate is genuine or is just telling you what you want to hear. So after it's all said and done, we look at some letters of recommendation (still waiting to see the first one where the candidate is not a superstar) before we make a calculated risk and offer the job.

The next ninety days of orientation and probation seem to go well...until it all falls apart on day ninety-one. We have all been there: How did he or she change, or why didn't I get that feeling when I was interviewing him or her?

The question is: How can we recruit for success?

Well, start off with knowing what you want and how you are going to support incoming candidates. Who is going measure productivity? When will you hold follow-up meetings, and how long should the probationary period be? Never hesitate to extend probation if any doubt exists. We have four basic principles that each candidate must have to some degree: *passion, skill, knowledge, and ability.* Never compromise on *passion*, though the others can vary to some extent. Next, would you buy a car without test-driving it first? Hell, no! Well, don't hire without testing or observing the candidates' passion, skills, knowledge, and ability.

Let them interact with your clients, organize a desk, or set up a project or PowerPoint. I have had folks request to go to the bathroom only to not return; they told me in the interview that they were expert users of Microsoft Office, but when it came time to complete a simple assignment, it was time to bail. You can design a short experiment for any discipline that will tell you more than any words on their résumés could. Actually, I don't even look at the résumés; if they can't tell their stories with passion, I'm no longer interested.

Chapter 22

Do You Have an Active Rerecruit Strategy?

Be honest with me for just a moment. How much time have you spent in the past year on rerecruitment of your staff? I imagine the vast majority of you are now scratching your heads and wondering what I even mean by *rerecruitment*.

As leaders on any level, we should not only be concerned about recruiting the *right* people for the *right* jobs, but we should be continuously on the lookout to find meaningful ways to engage, grow, and develop our high performers. After all, they are the most likely to leave and have a negative impact on our operations when they do.

Are you aware of the *cost* to recruit for a new position? It could be as much as a year's salary, especially when external recruiters are used. We also should know the time commitment to recruit, interview, get onboard, and orient new team members. When you start adding up the cost, loss of efficiency, continuity, and impact on other staff, rerecruitment of high performers is a much better proposition for your institution or business.

How do you rerecruit? Start simply by getting to know your staff members, what drives them, and what their one-, three-, and five-year personal-growth plans are. As a leader, you can become their coach and mentor to assist in career-goal development, creating opportunities to meet their intrinsic values and to provide realistic incentives that do not need to be monetary compensation at all times.

The fact that you spend extra quality time with high performers will allow you to continuously assess the likelihood of transition, which in turn will provide opportunities to set up a long-term transition plan to ensure minimal business impact on operations at large.

It is also your responsibility as a leader on any level to set clear professional goals for yourself and prepare your business unit for your departure by implementing succession planning.

Chapter 23

When Was the Last Time You Had Some Fun?

I always finish my interviews with new recruits by asking them what they do for *fun*. Try it yourself next time; it is truly revealing.

If someone asked me the same question, I would talk with pride about my flying escapades, which reveals something about me—not any different from someone who tells you he or she likes to knit, take photographs, hike, hunt, skydive, and so on.

It is essentially important to have fun in life; it can't all be about business. It's even better when you can combine working, learning, teaching, and developing into a fun activity.

Use creativity over capital; having *fun* doesn't have to be costly—just be innovative. If you are not an out-of-the box thinker, do a simple Google search and pick an idea from the hundreds of choices.

Some food for thought (no pun intended): cupcake wars, BBQ, or a "share a dish" event. There are also team-building exercises such as building a bridge, doing an egg drop, completing puzzles, and the like. If you have a few dollars available, there's the choice of bowling, a trip to local museums, or a concert. Remember the story about low performers? Maybe you can make one of them a party planner to reenergize and reengage him or her—just a thought.

Fun is relaxing, engaging, and necessary for us to stay sharp every day.

Plan something fun today for tomorrow.

Chapter 24

Why Team Building Is a Necessity

Pick a *team*, any *team*. Let's take Villanova, the NCAA champions. Did they become champions just because it was their turn, or was it earned through hard work, passion, and dedication to a common goal?

Of course the latter is where the magic took place; it all started with a crystal-clear goal that was articulated by the *team* leaders on day one: we are going all the way in 2016! I was not there, but I can hear the words coming out of the mouths of the coach, trainers, and team captains. Single focus, common understanding, common knowledge, and unwavering mutual respect with an open mind to learning and development are what led Villanova to become NCAA champions in 2016.

This magic needs to be translated to your business unit through *team* building. It all starts with finding the right focus and goals, followed by picking the right team members, who collectively buy in to the vision and strategy development by the team leaders and team members alike. No *team* has ever become champions overnight; most have struggled and learned along the way from many painful lessons but have survived and triumphed as a *team* because they believed in one another, made adjustments along the way, and were accountable to themselves and their team.

"What can I do today?" you should ask. Start by identifying what is most important for your business unit, then create the focus and vision around the process that is needed. Select key stakeholders who can drive the process to success (failure to include the *right* people will lead to failure and great frustration; it's like rolling a ball uphill). Form a *team* and start exercising together, to use a sports analogy. It's no different. There's more about teams and projects in later chapters.

Being a team is so much better than being a group.

Chapter 25

Loving Those You Lead

"Philia," as in Philadelphia, as in "City of Brotherly Love." How do you show love to your coworkers, direct reports, or loved ones? How does your boss show love toward you?

When was the last time you took the time to do something out of the ordinary to show some love toward those you lead? Most likely, it doesn't happen often enough, if at all.

Pause for a few minutes to reflect and self-assess. What makes you tick? How can you feel appreciated or respected in the work unit? Your personal answers are exactly that—unique to *you*; these are your intrinsic drivers.

As a leader on any level, it is your responsibility to figure out what each person's sweet spots are; we all have some. Some like to be rewarded with an extra day off or the opportunity to take the lead on a project, while the next person would appreciate a personalized thank-you card or the chance to be empowered to drive change in the organization.

Taking the time to *love* each person in his or her own way will make you and your business unit that much more successful. Make the time in your busy schedule; it's worth its weight in gold.

You can apply this in your personal relationships as well. I would recommend reading either *Five Languages of Love* or *Men Are from Mars, Women Are from Venus*. These books will teach you to interpret each other's language and make meaningful change in the way you express love to each other.

A healthy relationship at home will make you that much more effective at work.

Chapter 26

Laser Focus

Sit back, kick up your feet, scratch your chin, and make a mental list of all the projects you are currently working on—five, six, seven, or more. Now, assess honestly how well each project is going: Are you making progress, meeting your milestones, driving metrics toward your goals, or sustaining the improvements from your last completed projects?

I've got a feeling (the name of a song, I believe) that you are not meeting your targets and frequently end up backtracking to ensure sustainment of past improvements, which only impedes progress on your current projects.

The fact is that our behavioral capacity is limited. In other words, your ability to focus and be highly effective is limited to maybe two or three projects at any given time.

Even for the nonbelievers, try something different by working with *laser focus* over the next ninety days. Select a project that is aligned with your work unit's vision and strategic initiatives, that meets the threshold of significance, that has the bandwidth to be completed, and for which you have access to key stakeholders to succeed.

Keep in mind that to eat an elephant, you can do it *only* one bite at a time. Your focused project should be scoped for success with definable start and end points, including *SMART* metrics and goals.

Once you have all your ducks in a row, run your project using whatever process you have grown accustomed to, but set laser focus on thirty days for planning and measuring and sixty days to implement and sustain. I would almost bet you a dollar that your outcomes will meet or beat expectations for days, weeks, and months to come, as long as you continue to measure for at least another six months and take countermeasures when performance drops off.

Just because you focus on one project at a time, it doesn't mean you can't do anything else. Do what you do every day, but set aside enough time to have *laser focus* on a singular, major, impactful project that will drive success. Here's the equation:

Laser focus = 1–2 projects max; 3–5 might survive; >6 will die in place

Chapter 27

What to Do with Feedback

"Why do I need *feedback*? I'm perfect," said nobody ever!

Feedback is food for the professional soul; actually receiving structured feedback in a relationship of any kind is powerful, magical, and sometimes transformational.

One needs to be open to receive feedback; this requires a bit of courage and superior listening skills (receiving, processing, and pausing before responding). It's a heavy lift, especially for alpha-type leaders and staff members.

To be on a continuous journey of personal and professional growth, you need to receive feedback in many ways and from many different perspectives—male, female, peer, supervisor, or frontline staff member; each will provide valuable insights from which you can create opportunities. At times, it will bring you great validation; however, be mindful about whom and what motivates the person giving you that compliment.

Pure, honest, and critical feedback is what you seek. After receiving it, what should you do next?

Categorize feedback on a Pareto chart and use the 80/20 rule to decide what to work on next; include opportunities to strengthen and develop new skills and knowledge.

Most importantly, don't try fixing it all at once; identify the most meaningful, valuable, and attainable opportunity to work on first. It's important to create personal wins to build confidence and humility to work on the hard stuff.

Failure to do anything with feedback will lead to failure itself.

Feedback is food for your soul.

Chapter 28

Meaningful Metrics—Do You Agree?

Meaningfulness is in the eye of the beholder. Do we ever agree?

I daresay if you don't take the time to build consensus among stakeholders before you start measuring, nearly 100 percent of the time someone will claim the results are flawed and will be quick to blame the process of measuring as the reason *why* it's inaccurate or *why* a project didn't deliver desired outcomes.

Do yourself a big favor and very carefully include all *key* stakeholders to be part of designing the project, as well as selecting a meaningful metric. Meaningful metrics should be broken down into two categories:

- Driver metrics
- Outcome metrics

Each will be addressed separately under a different title, but one should understand and appreciate the need to have a solid foundation based on mutual respect, common understanding, and common goals among all key stakeholders.

Don't even bother if you don't have agreement; focus on consensus building around a metric that is measurable, reliable, meaningful, and aligned with your strategic vision.

Meaningful—is the metric going to give you information that will allow you to improve?

Chapter 29

Driver Metrics: What Are They?

No driver's license is required for this chapter, but if you're not careful, driver metrics will get away from you.

Let me set the stage by providing an analogy we can all relate to. You know that thing in your bathroom that you reluctantly stand on from time to time, and it always tells you what you don't want to know measured in pounds? Your scale will tell only your outcome metrics; however, if you want to *influence* that outcome, you need to concentrate on what makes your weight go up or down—in my case, more up than down!

Only once you pay attention to what goes in your mouth (this reminds me of a Dutch saying, "*Elk pondje gaat door het mondje*" [every pound gained must go through one's mouth]) can you start affecting the outcome.

Once you select a project and agree on a goal, you can work backward to find the right driver metric that will provide your team the ability to affect the outcome.

If your outcome metric is a fill rate of 85 percent, you can report on a weekly basis how you are performing against that goal. However, to affect the outcome, one needs to look at access slots, scheduling, templates, utilization, and so on. Each of these will drive the final outcome metric.

Not knowing what drives your metrics is like driving a car without a steering wheel.

Chapter 30

How Do Outcome Metrics Affect Us?

Get a box of tissues—most outcome metrics are tearjerkers, for goodness' or badness' sake.

In health care—or finance, for that matter—every time we look at a dashboard report, we are looking at nothing but outcome metrics. On their own, these metrics mean very little; however, against a benchmark, they will have an impact on some level.

Do you take the time to really understand both the measurement and the metric? Most of us don't; actually, most of us will shy away from metrics because we have a persistent allergy to mathematics that even fifty milligrams of Benadryl can't suppress.

Let's take a step backward. You are starting a new project. The first question is *why* did you select this project, based on *what*? A regulatory mandate? Did the boss wake up on the wrong side of the bed? Or is the project strategically aligned with your company's vision or best-practice standard that you would like to adopt for yourself?

Now that you have sorted out why you are starting a new project, all key stakeholders should agree on the desired *outcome*. This can come from a national benchmark or simply may be picked by your leadership team. I would suggest you always use *SMART* as your guide to select the right outcome and driver metrics. Once selected, you can start monitoring for improvement.

If you're wondering how outcome metrics affect you, I will say the following:

They will make you smile or cry, but that's about it. The magic is in the driver metrics.

Chapter 31

Crucial to Create Wins for the Team

How would you feel if you were playing in a baseball game and the umpire removed home plate, preventing either team from scoring any runs? Most would not tolerate that for very long and would feel uninspired to continue playing.

Win or *lose*, we feel engaged and inspired.

Kick your feet up again, hang your head back in a relaxing position, and mentally assess whether your teams are set up to win anything. Do they have realistic and attainable goals for their projects? Do you have the right driver and outcome metrics in place? When was the last time you celebrated a win? How did your team *feel* after a win?

OK, now get your feet off my furniture.

If you've determined that your staff is pretty uninspired, it's very likely that they can't create a *win*. If that's the case, it's time to change up the game.

To create a win, I would suggest you include staff members who are going to be affected by the win to select the parameters, scope, and metrics for your project or process. You may even consider selecting the *right* reward for creating a *win*.

Money is not the first or second intrinsic driver for most of your staff members to create wins; recognition of the team or individuals is most important, although a little pizza party never hurts either!

Teams need to feel inspired, and nothing does the job better than creating a win.

Big or small accomplishments, we all like to be winners.

Chapter 32

Connecting the Dots

Do you ever feel like you are working with no end in sight or are all over the place without making any progress that can be either seen or felt?

We have all been on that wild-goose chase, only to never catch up and make the kill. It's like chasing your own tail—looks like fun, but it's dizzying, to say the least. At the end of the day, you feel unfulfilled, deflated, and at times disengaged.

Leading through context and connecting the dots are building blocks that can't be skipped over; it's like building a house of cards with a shaky foundation. Your strategic vision needs to make sense to those you lead. Your job as a leader is to align all efforts to meet or exceed the vision's expectations.

There are two essential steps to improving successful outcomes:

Step one

Take the time to clearly articulate the vision and put it into a real context. Depending on your audience, you may have to go into the weeds a bit; get this right before you go to step two.

Step two

Involve all key stakeholders in this step. Brainstorm potential solutions and pathways to get the desired outcomes. Next, be truly diligent about aligning your work—what comes first, second, third, and so on. By connecting the dots in a way that frontline personnel can understand, engagement with what you are trying to accomplish as a team will improve significantly.

Visual management tools that allow all involved to see progress made toward a common goal are not only powerful communication tools but are also key drivers to successful completion.

Connect the dots, and you will improve success.

Chapter 33

Staying on Top—Read a Lot

Does that leadership book come with cartoon pictures and extra-large letters?

We all know the traditional pathway to get to the top: high school, college degree(s), and maybe a certificate or two. But then what? All that was traditional, theoretical learning and little to do with what I'm doing now.

No matter what stage of your career you are in, you are not staying at the top or getting to the next level by doing little; it takes a lot of passion, energy, and time to rise to the top—and even more to *stay* there.

Reading industry-specific publications is an essential habit to form, not only to stay up-to-date with current affairs but also to identify opportunities to capture market space, advancement in technology, or ways to improve systems.

If you are serious about your career, you should belong to industry-specific professional associations and read their publications regularly. You should also add the best in business magazines, hardcovers, and web-based articles to your reading repertoire.

Be informed; stay informed. This is the most frequently asked question I get about this chapter: When do you have time to read? Make it a priority to read at work. Schedule a fake meeting on your calendar to create some *me* time. Turn off your computer and rummage through your trade magazines.

Heavier reading should be reserved for later in the day. Actually, if your commute is more than thirty minutes, books on tape are a great way to stay informed.

Here's a word of caution: we have all done this, especially after we come back from conferences, but don't change just because your latest book offered you a great technique or practice. Absorb what you read and understand the best practices and how they would affect your organization or work group. Involve or share your readings with your teammates, followed by a discussion about possible changes.

Read a lot to stay on top.

Chapter 34

Are You a Change Agent?

I always thought change agents rotated furniture in waiting rooms! Actually, a *change agent* is a person from inside or outside an organization who helps the organization transform itself by focusing on such matters as organizational effectiveness, improvement, and development.

Now that we've cleared the air, are *you* a change agent?

By function alone, you are someone who is striving to make processes more effective—of course, the minimum competency of a leader is to improve and develop.

Still, the question remains: Are you an effective change agent?

How can you be effective if you have not studied, participated, facilitated, or simply observed other change agents? We can all bring about *change*; however, only few are truly effective as change agents. For example, if you are changing processes that are not relevant to overall vision and strategic objectives, you are not effectively using your time or that of your teammates; therefore, you are not a change agent.

To effect change, you need to be in alignment with overall strategic objectives. Process changes should directly contribute to the larger outcome metric. To be a change agent, there's no need to change the world; however, your improvements *should* affect vision.

Would you like to be a change agent? If so, follow a couple of simple rules: develop a good understanding of your mission, vision, and value statement; identify areas of opportunities that are in direct alignment with mission, vision, and value; and study the change-agent tools, such as LEAN, Six Sigma, PDCA, TQM, FMEA, or RCA. Scope the project appropriately with clear ins and outs. Include all stakeholders in the process change. Plan, improve, implement, and sustain.

Be the change you want to see.

Chapter 35

Transformation to Stay Ahead

The days of slow evolution—like the African elephants growing their ears to stay cool over thousands of years—are long behind us. Or are they?

If you are not convinced that we need change measured in days or weeks, not decades or centuries, call the budget office in Washington, DC, and inquire what percentage of the GDP is dedicated to health-care expenses. If they answer you, inquire about its trajectory. Change alone is not good enough to ensure economic viability; we need transformation!

This means profound and radical change that orients an organization in a new direction and takes it to an entirely different level of effectiveness.

As a leader, you need to learn to think outside the box; otherwise, you will just make changes and not meet the need to transform.

Let me give you a brief exercise to see if you have what it takes (see the dot exercise in the appendix on team building). Connect the dots with only four straight lines; the lines can't cross over one another on any dot. The only hint I will give you is that it takes out-of-the-box thinking to solve this dilemma.

With certainty, I can tell you that today's business problems, especially those we face in health care at large, will require transformation with a great sense of urgency.

Be bold and brave.

Chapter 36

Stagnation Will Lead to Disaster

What happens with a swimming pool that sits without chemicals or a running filtration system for a couple of months? It goes from pure joy to a cesspool of danger. Is this any different from a department that is not innovating, developing, changing, or transforming with the times? People, places, or things that become stagnant are doomed to be left behind.

This should be enough for leaders to feel stimulated and strive for continuous development and improvement in their areas of operations.

As leaders on any level of the organization, we are responsible not only for driving change and transformation by leading through vision, energy, and passion but also for being hyperaware of stagnation within subdivisions—and even down to individuals.

To use my pool as an example, once bacteria or algae are established, they will spread until they are confronted and mitigated. This is no different from a manager who is stuck in the past, micromanages, prevents innovation beyond self, and relies on being directive. That managerial style needs to be confronted before it's too late.

The root cause is frequently lack of skill and ability in the individual and failure to be developed by his or her leader. It is extremely likely that the offenders are not aware of their stagnation and can recover once confronted.

Go back and reread my chapter on feedback. Create a safe environment, tell the staff member something positive, and explain to him or her how his or her behavior is affecting the operations. Listen carefully to his or her response and set crystal-clear expectations that can be monitored and measured for impact. Most importantly, follow up with the staff member regularly to ensure success.

Get rid of stagnation and turn it into gold.

Chapter 37

How Do You Work with Unions?

How does that saying go? Keep your friends close but your enemies closer. This has been the traditional mind-set for way too long. I have never understood *why* we fight with our unions. Why not embrace them instead?

My basic principles of effective management are mutual respect, common bond, common understanding, and teachability.

Keeping this in mind, can we agree that union bosses want to have a growing base of members and employers want highly qualified and engaged staff?

Why not agree that we want highly qualified contributing staff members and that we will replace every displaced staffer with another staffer? This would assure the union that its base remains the same or is growing and employers that you will replace low-performing staff members.

It sounds oversimplified, but really it all starts with relationship building and a hard reset on all sides of the equation.

Leaders should embrace a strong relationship with their unions and meet weekly to involve them in every aspect of governance and system improvements. It is vital that leaders and representatives of both sides develop a common bond and understanding. Only once you agree to be transparent and set common goals can you forge forward with objectives that are mutually beneficial.

Sounds dreamy, right? Not so quick!

I have had a deep, personal experience with both NYSNA and SIEU 1199. We worked together on complex issues and came up with mutually agreed-upon solutions without major conflict simply because we adhered to the two most important principles: *mutual respect* and *teachability*.

Give it a try—there's nothing to lose and everything to gain.

Chapter 38

Building Bridges between Key Stakeholders

As much as I dislike sitting on the Tappan Zee Bridge every morning, it's a true privilege and likely a once-in-a-lifetime experience to see a bridge-building project. See? My glass is always half-full.

Working within your circle of influence is always a bit easier than having to reach out to external departments, leaders, or staff members not directly under your influence.

Not unlike a soccer team, defense has to communicate with offense and coordinate efforts to ensure success both on defensive and offensive ends of the field.

In your work unit, it's unlikely that you have direct control over functions such as information technology or support services but see them as essential partners to overall success. Therefore, it is imperative to build bridges between departments as soon as possible—I mean *strong, nimble, bidirectional* bridges that will last over time.

Depending on the behavioral capacity of your counterparts and you, you may have to assess WIFM 101 ("what's in it for me?") and develop a common bond or understanding.

Be mindful to build bridges on the right level of the organization and include the right key stakeholders. Failure to assess and adjust will cost you time, political capital, and value at the back end.

Lead through context, not by directives.

Chapter 39

Do You Have a Bully in the Workplace?

We have all worked with incompetent coworkers and leaders who bully their way through their days and, sad to say, at times to the top of the organizational chart.

The last time I checked, it's 2016, and this type of behavior should no longer be tolerated in the workplace, especially not as a way of managing anything.

Most often, both the bully and his or her leaders lack the behavioral capacity to address this kind of operational style, which is detrimental to both service excellence and the financial sustainability of the organization.

We need to stand up against workplace violence of any kind and should not tolerate suppression, depression, defamation, or anything else that does not meet the ethical standards of service excellence in your organization.

Ask why bullies get away with this behavior. It's simple: it's ignored and rarely addressed. From personal experience, I believe most bullies don't see what we see and therefore can't or won't make adjustments because they are blinded to their own behaviors. Once addressed and exposed, most will make drastic changes, and others will soon leave or should be facilitated in leaving the organization.

Bullies are consistent in their behavior; it's the only way they know how to operate. They lack the skill, knowledge, and ability to conform to being a collaborative and servant leader.

It's time to roll up your sleeves, address the bully, and work side by side to coach or mentor him or her for success.

Chapter 40

Are You Really Listening?

Why did God give us two ears and one mouth? God's message to us all is to listen twice as much as we speak.

I've certainly been guilty of not doing that over the years. In my feedback sessions, I have been called a fire hydrant, have had it suggested to me that less is more, and have been told a few times to shut up and listen.

Very few of us are actual accomplished listeners; most of us don't even understand how to really listen when spoken to. Think back for a moment to an intense conversation; while someone was speaking and you were supposed to be listening, you likely were already very busy formulating a response, precluding you from really listening.

There are three phases of listening that we need to appreciate and exercise before ever becoming an active listener: *receiving, processing,* and *responding.*

Each phase requires additional study, which we can't cover in just one short chapter; however, I would recommend that you take the time to explore this further. Since most of you won't take the time, here're my two cents on becoming a better listener.

Remove yourself from all distractions: computers, phones, and televisions. Sit together at a table and not behind your desk.

Quality over Quantity

Most importantly, process information received before even starting to formulate a response. You even want to repeat what you think you heard; this will buy you some time as well as confirm that you actually heard what you were listening to.

Practice makes perfect. This is much harder than you think, but you can do it.

Chapter 41

Are You Committed to Improving Every Day?

What did you do today that made a difference for tomorrow? Are you committed like a pig is to an egg-and-bacon sandwich or merely engaged, like the chicken?

Of course, improving something every day can come in many ways, such as process improvement, projects, relationship building, professional development, or personal enhancements.

Being committed to improving speaks to a certain mind-set rather than to an actual outcome on a daily basis. If you are passionate and energetic each time you walk into your workplace, acknowledging coworkers with a friendly smile and genuine "good morning," you most likely have met the threshold of improving something that day.

Being committed to improving means you are teachable and willing to receive constructive feedback from which to improve. Being committed to improving means you are willing to share experiences, teach, and develop your staff on any given day. Improving every day is really living life to its fullest extent.

Now that you are committed to improving, as a pig is committed to providing bacon to a delicious sandwich, start your day by embracing the opportunity to make a difference by simply saying the following:

"Good morning. How are you today?"

Chapter 42

Everything We Do Is Just Another Process

Even brushing your teeth is a process that can be done right, wrong, or not at all. Each of these options has a consequence—good, bad, or indifferent.

Men especially love to jump to conclusions, skipping necessary process steps to put in place solutions that likely will come back to haunt us later.

Getting each process right will save lives, increase margins, improve quality, reduce error rates, and ensure our workplaces are safe.

It is absolutely necessary to learn a basic quality tool, such as process mapping, before you can start identifying process gaps or hold discussions about solutions. Each workflow has multiple process steps that must be aligned and sequenced to ensure fluency and flow.

Let's go back to brushing your teeth. How many processes can you identify?

- Have toothpaste and toothbrush.
- Put toothpaste on toothbrush.
- Brush lower teeth.
- Brush upper teeth.
- Rinse.
- Clean toothbrush.

Each process has subprocess steps that you'll need to document; only after you identify each step can you find the root cause that can lead to potential outcomes, such as having the wrong toothpaste, wrong brush, or wrong technique—or maybe even how you rinse and clean your brush.

Chapter 43

Haunted by Policies

Having buyer's regret? Has a regulatory agency ever cited you for violating your own policies? There's nothing worse, but does it happen all the time?

Let's be honest—when was the last time you looked at your policy and procedure manuals? Most are collecting dust on a lonely shelf or stuck in the digital world, waiting for some attention every two to three years.

We are indeed haunted by our own policies. All too frequently, adjustments are made to processes without our updating our own manuals. It's like chasing Bigfoot in the Adirondacks.

We need to stop generating so many policies that just sit on a shelf; instead, we should generate an operations manual and treat it like a living document where we post standard work practices.

We should consolidate as many policies as possible to streamline our maintenance requirements and reduce the risk that these policies overstate what is actually taking place on the ground.

So instead of living in a haunted house, create a living document with operational guidelines and best practices. Show clear documentation that information was shared to all staff and check back frequently to ensure that information is accurate. Don't let the creep set in; looking at P&Ps every three years is not the recommended route to ensure compliance.

In the case of policies, we need to underpromise and overdeliver.

Chapter 44

Regulations: Guardrail versus Guide Rail

Somebody once told me a story about the difference between a guardrail and a guide rail. Of course, the story involved an "ambulance-chasing lawyer" to define the difference.

Once upon a time, the New York State Department of Transportation referred to those metal things along the road as guardrails…until some slick law firm sued them, claiming their client wasn't protected by the guardrail as he flipped his car over the side of a cliff. Ever since, the New York State Department of Transportation has been referring to those metal things on the side of the road as *guide rails*.

There's a powerful lesson to be learned for all of us: protocols or policies are not guardrails. They guide us through processes by suggesting best practices, but they still leave room for us to think and adjust as scenarios change along the way. They do not guard us from harm when ignored or violated.

Protocols and policies will protect you only when you can justify the action. Simply said, they guide you through a process based on actual data that supports a regulation or mandate that will set you up for quality, safety, and successful outcomes.

Regulations are a necessary evil in today's very litigious society, but keep in mind that only you can decide right from wrong.

Be a great carpenter by measuring twice and cutting once. Ask the questions that need to be asked.

Chapter 45

Are We Still Allowed to Use Our Common Sense?

Oh, no...being practical, pragmatic, and free to think for ourselves! In some business units, this will get you in trouble quicker than doing much of nothing.

Complacency will creep into any organization when you don't allow your talented staff to be creative, be involved, or be empowered. Too many directive leaders will try to micromanage every minute detail in their operations and will see common sense as something dangerous in the workplace.

It starts by recognizing your own leadership style on any level of the organization. Are you passive, passive-aggressive, a delegator, directive, supportive, an enabler, a servant, or collaborative, just to mention a few?

What we do know is that leaders who are collaborative and servants will empower their staffs to take part of every decision-making process and provide the freedom to make commonsense decisions and solutions on the spot, as long as they are willing to learn from their mistakes and understand when to share or consult and seek assistance before a decision is made.

What can you do today? Let go by appreciating the fact that we learn more from our failures than we will ever realize. Most often, common sense prevails, and your staff will be more engaged than they would be if you took the directive route of managing.

Unlock the magic in your staff; empower them to be sensible and pragmatic.

Chapter 46

Risk Mitigation

What is the most common reaction after the fact? "Oops, if we had only..."

Be honest—that is frequently the reaction to process failures: "If we had only stopped talking and done something about it." You know the cost of mitigation versus reaction and fallout cost? I don't, and I don't *want* to know. All I know is that it's always far more expensive to react to something than to be proactive.

Risk mitigation is just as valid in patient care as it is in emergency management or business operations. Connect the dots to any disaster, and you will find that you had opportunities to prevent, mitigate, or be prepared to respond.

Why do we fail so badly? Partly because we suffer from syndromes called "that will never happen to me"—"I can't afford prevention," or "I'm too busy or lazy."

Risk mitigation should be a center point of your business plan, whether your business is health care, finance, or IT solutions. You really can't afford not to do this. Buying extra insurance is not a solution. Great leaders will perform regular *failure-mode effect analysis* to determine at-risk areas and will work diligently to reduce financial and public exposure.

In health care, we are required by law to have a robust emergency-management plan, including an annual *hazard-vulnerability analysis,* which mandates that we have some planning, mitigation, and response plans in place for the top three to five likeliest scenarios.

Each of you should perform a mini FMEA in your work unit and have a basic preparedness plan for workforce replacement or making sure you have electricity in your office during an outage. Thinking about it when responding to an emergency is a bit too late.

An ounce of prevention is worth its weight in gold. Don't delay; mitigate risk today.

Chapter 47

Do You Know the Cost of Everything?

Let's have a moment of honesty among friends. Have you ever gone into a supply room to grab two or three items, knowing full well that you needed only one? Have you ever taken something home from your workplace, such as paper supplies, pens, and so on? I know you have, because I have been watching you!

Let's use an example to drive the point home. As a team, we worked diligently to set up a reprocessing program to reduce both waste and cost for our surgical program. One of the items we identified was surgical staples. Once we started exploring opportunities, we noticed that rarely were more than ten staples ever used out of the thirty available. So we thought we were slick and replaced all surgical staplers with ones that hold only ten. We were proud of ourselves for bringing significant savings to our program; however, reality set in quickly when we noticed that surgeons now took three staplers into the operating room, causing the same waste at a higher cost.

Are you scratching your head yet? What did we do wrong? It made sense to us—but not to them. Their old behavior carried over to our revamped program. What did we miss? We included their leaders in the discussion, agreed on the new product line, and informed our staff. It seems like we followed all the basic principles of good project management.

Did you get it yet? We didn't highlight the cost of each item and how much it would save or what we could purchase if we saved. Only once we started labeling the cost of everything from four-by-four alcohol wipes to surgical staplers and so on did we start saving significantly, and even theft (another term for permanent borrowing) across the board diminished.

What's the moral of this short story? Put value (cost) on everything, if at all possible. Frontline staffers should know what these things cost and contribute to the bottom line.

Once your team members understand the cost, their subconscious will be more conscientious about waste.

Chapter 48

Complacency—Old versus New

Complacency is what brings airplanes down with wheels up and wings down.

Complacency in its simplest definition means a feeling of being satisfied with how things are and not wanting to try to make them better: a complacent feeling or condition.

Complacency can be due to success or failure to thrive. Complacency can be related to a person or an organization. The common thread is the fact that things are being taken for granted. At times, innovation slows after a big win or when folks have nothing to play for any longer; there's a lost sense of urgency or ability to win, or teams have simply lost the love and are now just passing time.

Complacency is almost always the fault of poor leadership.

Complacency is like bacteria that won't go away, especially if you take only three days' worth of antibiotics while the prescription clearly states ten days. Complacency will fester until it is eradicated.

Old complacency comes from comfort or lack of inspiration and accountability. New complacency comes from taking things for granted and having expectations. Regardless of old or new, leaders need to find ways to stimulate old minds and show new minds the finer touches of life itself. Start living in the moment, stimulate, originate, and be the change you want to see.

As a *positude* leader, your mission is to be a visionary to all generations and lead through context in a shared and collaborative environment. Be on the lookout for the team members who no longer smile or look up to greet you when you come in.

Create a safe environment and discuss with your team members ways to be reengaged in the workplace. Stimulate their behavioral capacity by providing stimulating and passionate leadership.

Break bad habits before they become the new norm.

Chapter 49

It All Starts with Trust

Trust is the foundation of *respect*; without it, there's not much to go on. Whether one has to earn respect to receive respect is an age-old question, but isn't that essentially the same question as "What came first, the *chicken* or the *egg*?"

Frequently, respect, or lack thereof, is the number-one cited barrier to success and performance in any organization. One's feelings, insights, and contributions are not valued, which is often expressed as "I'm not trusted or respected."

I'm a believer that you show respect to all and translate trust into empowerment under the rules of validation and verification.

If you adopt a nonjudgmental approach to managing, plus a strong coaching and mentoring model, your staff will feel a sense of security around making decisions and asking questions without being blamed or punished when unmalicious failures occur.

Trust is an important ingredient to long-term relationships, whether personal or professional. Success takes ongoing efforts and strong communication skills to ensure satisfaction and productivity.

As a leader, manager, supervisor, or frontline staff member, show respect to all in the most simplistic ways, such as acknowledgment and being grateful for whatever team members contribute to the bottom line. Make a real effort to develop a common bond and understanding in regard to expectations.

One who gives is more likely to receive.

Chapter 50

Partnering with Adversaries

There are three types of bosses: those who take, those who give, and those who are incompetent.

It's the incompetent adversarial boss you need to be mindful of and depart from as soon as is practically possible.

A *taking* adversarial boss is in it for him- or herself; however, those individuals will support you to some extent to ensure self-success. They readily take all the credit from any project that was successful and suppress failures. If you love what you do and get gratification from your contributions, you can survive and, when the timing is right, succeed. Make sure the balance is in your favor in regard to learning and professional-growth perspective.

The incompetent bosses will take all credit and place blame on others for their failures. They are the absolute worst takers. They are most often tightly connected to senior managers who frequently will turn a blind eye to sheer incompetence as long as quality and safety are not compromised. Extract yourself as soon as possible. Under this kind of leadership, you will be suppressed instead of developed. There is no compromise or ability to negotiate, due either to lack of intellectual ability or fear of smarter people working for them.

To maintain a positive outlook and receive the professional support you deserve, seek alternatives.

To those considering a new role, *always* ask about professional development, coaching, and mentoring programs. I would also reach out to some current staffers to assess leadership style and follow through with offered programs.

As a *positude* leader, I'm always searching for a giver and recommend you do the same.

A leopard doesn't change its spots.

Chapter 51

If It Were Only That Simple—Cut the Bottom 10 Percent

Jack Welch once said that cutting the bottom 10 percent of your workforce several years in a row will get you a performance team the quickest. This is sad but true. This is easy to say and, for most of us, very difficult to execute, for a variety of reasons.

Those working in union environments will run into resistance that will take years to overcome, especially if they were to figure out that you plan to cut the bottom 10 percent year after year.

Others would like to cut the bottom 10 percent; however, they don't have access to a labor pool to replace lost workers with ones that meet their expectations.

What do you do now that you are stuck between a rock and a hard place?

We need to deploy some common sense and perform a top-down and bottom-up assessment of our workforce, utilizing our basic four principles to score performance as high, middle, or low: *passion, knowledge, skill,* and *ability*.

What you should see appearing is a natural bell curve that identifies those in *low* and *middle* sectors in need of remediation and those in *high* sectors, who are deserving of rerecruitment.

Start with the staff members with very low *passion* scores. Work with them individually to find why they are not engaged; work together to find common grounds to reignite their passion from within. Most will be successful.

Since most of us are not in the position to just slash and burn, we need to use our leadership skills, especially our coaching and mentoring, and as my son Max often says, we need to be part-time therapists.

Don't give up on your bottom 10 percent until the time is truly right.

Chapter 52

Does Culture Really Eat Strategy for Breakfast?

Culture would like to have stack of pancakes with three eggs over easy, whole-wheat toast, and strawberry jelly with a little strategy on the side. Yum...I'm actually getting hungry!

What is the difference between *culture* and *strategy*?

Let's take a brief look at both to see if culture really eats strategy for breakfast.

Where does culture come from? Can it be imposed on us or taught to us? Should we even be involved in culture development, or is it someone else's job?

Culture needs to come from within and be aligned with your company's vision—first as an individual, then as a team, and lastly as the entire organization—before one can say you have a culture that is aligned. Most importantly, *culture* is *always* an activity or feeling, not just when you feel like it. You can self-assess where your organization currently is.

Strategy is the *way* your organization is going to meet expectations set by the *vision*. There are many roads that lead to Rome, as they say. Even a lousy strategy can produce results, as well as poor organizational culture; however, to get top performance, all three need to be in alignment:

$$(Culture)(Strategy) > Vision\ Performance\ Indicators$$

To exceed expectations through strong performance, each individual in the organization needs to understand his or her contributions and relevance to the outcomes he or she seeks.

Culture will eat strategy for breakfast, lunch, *and* dinner; therefore, as leaders, it is our responsibility to lead our teams to define culture on the local level and hold all stakeholders accountable always.

Culture must start from within each individual, led by example.

Chapter 53

Only When You Change the Game

Einstein, one of the wisest men of our ages, is believed to have said, "The definition of insanity is doing the same thing over and over and expecting a different outcome."

How often do you see this around you? Needless to say, you have never participated in or led such an activity, right? It's like a gambler who goes back to the casino night after night and only wins; at least, that's what he says, but we all know better.

The real question is: Why do we participate in such insane activities, knowing that the outcome is going to be a variable of the same? It's our behavior against or unwillingness to be different or to take a risk that prevents us from changing our approaches.

If you are not convinced, read the first thirty pages of *Change the Culture, Change the Game* to see the results once a brave leader takes charge and breaks the perpetual cycle of insanity.

Results are not guaranteed, but failure to *change the game* will lead to eventual disaster. Therefore, the alternative holds true—you might as well change the game and go down in flames if it fails to make the difference. I'm not recommending this; however, it does sound interesting.

What I do recommend is for you to assemble your team and clearly spell out the current state of affairs to gain understanding. What has gone wrong that has landed you in this current state? Next, identify go-to leaders within your department, and start by challenging them to think differently and out of the box to come up with a new strategy for performance.

Encourage creativity, and empower them to find sustainable solutions. It will be amazing to see what has been harbored within your talented staff but has gone untapped until now.

Change the culture, change the game.

Chapter 54

Are We Huddling Enough?

We have heard it all: "Another huddle" frequently goes hand-in-hand with "Do we really have to huddle?" And "Can we huddle later?" is the companion to "Not everybody is here, so we can cancel the huddle," and "We don't huddle on weekends!"

Anyone who expresses one of the statements above—or a variation of them—clearly doesn't understand the purpose of the huddle at large. Let's discuss the need to huddle before assessing if we huddle enough.

When pilots prepare for a cross-country flight or surgeons prepare for an amputation, what is the minimum expected to be done prior to starting the engines or introducing an anesthetic? A flight briefing and time-out—both have saved many planes from crashing and wrong limbs from being cut off; mistakes would be costly if they were to happen due to skipping these simple steps to ensure *safety* and *quality*.

How does this relate to huddles? Well, as communication failures are our top three reasons for process failures that lead to poor outcomes, setting up a reliable communication protocol is the desired and sustainable solution to mitigate such circumstances.

Therefore, huddles actually can be interpreted as a meaningful way of communicating, whereby we deploy techniques such as *ask-tell-ask* or *read back and verify*. This will ensure that all three phases of active listening are engaged: *receiving*, *processing*, and *responding*.

To go back to the original question—"Are we huddling enough?"—the answer is most likely not. Most still don't see the real value in huddling or even taking a time-out in an operating theater. As a leader, you must lead through context and find the value proposition to engage all staff in huddles and not make them dependent on any one individual or process.

Huddling = Communications = Quality and Safety

Chapter 55

Is There Anything More Important Than Quality?

I would ask that question of a nuclear-power-plant operator who may produce the highest quality of energy but die in the process of delivering a quality product. Quality is important, but it always needs to be evaluated in the context of safety, not just on its own.

The overarching responsibility of the board and president or CEO of any organization is to ensure quality in a safe work environment.

Coming from a Six Sigma quality-control background, I learned a while back that variation is the silent killer of quality. We need to measure all phases of production to ensure a quality product or process at the end. Remember the conversation about driver metrics and outcome metrics? They are an absolute must-have when we discuss quality.

Setting safety to the side for just a minute, quality mandates tight upper and lower control limits to observe variation that could lead to poor quality outcomes. In our fancy world of computers, leaders prefer that you electronically measure and be warned when either limit is violated. Especially in health care, quality is linked to applying best practices to procedures such as central-line insertion and prevention of wrong-sided surgeries; therefore, human observations are necessary to ensure consistency with every process.

Let's get safety back on the couch for another joint counseling session with quality. We should never separate them again; you can't have quality without safety or safety without quality—happily married, after all, for life!

Quality and safety are synonymous with *top priority*.

Cut corners, and it will get you every time.

Chapter 56

Political Capital: How to Spend Your PC Money

'Tis the season for political capital to be gained and reserved for future usage...or is it? Don't we always complain about those damn politicians who take money from large corporations and powerful lobbyists only to be beholden to them once in office?

The game we all despise so much is precisely the tactic you can use in your workplace to get things done. I'm only advocating above-the-line transactions and condemn any below-the-line activities—no brown-paper baggies filled with goodies for me!

Actually, if you go back in time, *trading* was a very acceptable term for a transaction taking place between two people. Living "innatura" is based on trade rather than on exchange of money.

Let's get back to our topic of political capital and how you can spend it. Since a *positude* leader is a proactive, go-to positive leader in the organization, you will frequently find yourself assisting others with removal of barriers to their success. Each time you get such an opportunity, you are actually building up some PC cash. Be smart about it. Show appreciation for the opportunity to assist, and look forward to working with them in the future.

Sooner or later, your PC cash will come in handy to remove a barrier for your team without having to compromise or wait till it is your turn in the rotation. Word of caution: Put your PC cash to work at the right time with the right people. Don't waste it on folks who are in your corner already. Use it to overcome a natural barrier or personality in your organization.

Be a gracious giver and a tactful taker.

Chapter 57

Can We Convert Naysayers?

Over the years, I have had the opportunity to work with some real characters, but none stand out more than the ones who are persistently negative. Pure negativity is one of the only things that get my blood boiling, and I have to be constantly aware to prevent a nuclear meltdown.

We all have experienced this throughout our professional careers. There are two types of personalities we won't forget soon: there's always someone who has done, seen, or experienced every possible scenario, and there's always someone who starts off with "That's not going to work." My blood is starting to boil—time for some cold water!

Without going into the psychology of negativity, can we break this cycle and regain some sense of normalcy with perpetual naysayers?

I believe these types of personalities are no different from an LP needle being stuck on the same track; after a while, it is their new norm—a bad norm, may I say.

After years of operating from that side of the brain, it will take a hard reset to get them back on track. This is where your leadership and behavioral capacity come to task. The naysayer most likely is not aware of his or her own negativity until somebody works up the courage to provide critical feedback, not by placing blame but rather by showing this person the impact of his or her attitude on teammates and his or her limits on creativity.

Having this conversation will be the first step in the naysayer's recovery—not perfection.

Don't give up on the ol' LP yet. For you millennials, Google long-playing record! Often all it takes is a little nudge.

Chapter 58

Are You Really Committed?

Should I repeat the story of the pig's role in the bacon-and-egg sandwich? Nah, you get it—unless, of course, you are not committed to reading my book and landed on this page by accident.

Just to make sure, I'm not alluding to your being committed to the local psych ward either!

Let's use a real scenario all of you have experienced. You have been assigned a project that crosses over multiple departments and has a tight deadline. This is your opportunity to rise to the occasion and deliver for your boss. Time to shine. We have all been there, right? Next is selecting the right teammates and setting up the project, including key milestones and weekly meeting schedules to gauge progress. Sound familiar?

Next is the difference between someone who's committed to your project—such as you—versus someone who is merely engaged. This is likely somebody outside of your immediate work group.

After a few weeks, you have scheduled the first follow-up meeting to review progress toward upcoming milestones. You are ready to go before you get an e-mail from one of your critical teammates requesting a change in the meeting time or date due to another conflict on the schedule, only to find out he or she had a hot lunch date. Needless to say, at the next meeting, he or she was ill-prepared and didn't meet deliverables as requested.

The real question should be whether you're able to find teammates who will be committed to your project before you get started.

As a leader, it is essential that you perform your due diligence in selecting the right people for the right roles to improve your chances of success. You need to select coworkers who understand and share common goals to improve success rates. Their value proposition needs to be aligned with yours. If they are not aligned, you likely will end up with noncompliant teammates or, at times, even some saboteurs.

The golden rule for commitment is this: right roles, right people.

Chapter 59

Tolerance

As a leader, you will be representing a small or, at times, large group of staff members from diverse backgrounds, some of whom likely live an alternate lifestyle. As a great leader, you should be tolerant and supportive without hesitation to ensure equality across the board. Sadly, I have experienced otherwise and have seen too many lives lost due to suicide. This is a message from my heart with hope that it will make a difference to someone somewhere.

Tolerance—why is it so difficult to be accepting of all human beings and their chosen lifestyles? Why is it still so difficult for self-identified LGBTQ members to come out and be proud? The short answer is lack of tolerance from parents, brothers, sisters, teachers, religion, and society at large.

How many more kids need to take their own lives before we answer the question by simply loving the individual and showing compassion and tolerance?

Let's work together to make a difference and live without regret. Reach-out Wednesday (ROW) is a great way to reach out and touch a life that needs to be shown love and compassion.

Those most vulnerable are the ones still searching for the courage to step forward and be proud publicly. For them, we need to tone down the rhetoric and be more supportive in our public statements.

Open your arms to all God's children, and provide them with the security to live life to its fullest potential.

Tolerance and love are powerful tools in suicide prevention. Come ROW with me!

Chapter 60

Living in the Now

As I drove from Burlington, Vermont, back to my home in New City, New York, it could have been just another long ride of thinking about the days ahead of me or listening to the kids pestering one another. Instead, I tried to enjoy every mile and minute that went by, looking at the beauty of our surroundings, particularly as everything was starting to come alive again.

From the mountains in the far distance to the weathered barns along the way, each landmark has a story to tell; however, we rarely take the time to listen. We are missing out on so much because we fail ourselves by thinking about tomorrow while *now* slips away into history.

Today, for many hours on end, I tried my darnedest to stay in the now by observing the little things along the way and not allowing my mind to drift into the tomorrow. I noticed the blossoms on apple trees, calves in their outdoor pans, grass growing, and birds flying north. I observed the changing weather patterns and the fact that only a few hundred miles is the difference between bare trees and those in full green. I enjoyed the sounds of children playing in the backseat and appreciated the cute comments from my son Max and daughter Maia.

Today, I realized how lucky I really am. Living in the moment, living in the now, is worth everything to me.

Chapter 61

What to Do with a Saboteur

Whenever I hear the word *saboteur*, I think back to World War II stories from my father and mother. Saboteurs worked with Nazis to fight the Dutch resistance and identify homes where Jews were hidden from capture.

In every sense of the word, I despise what it means, but I acknowledge that they are not only among us but within us.

Being a positive leader leaves you vulnerable to attack from saboteurs who will prey on your natural naïveté. As a *positude* leader, your natural position will be to trust until proven otherwise. As a positive leader, you will need to grow some eyes in the back of your head to hold off the negative forces that look to derail you whenever they can.

This sounds dramatic, but it's true. The higher you go up the administrative career ladder, the larger the crowd eyeing your job.

If that is not enough, you need to be conscious of your inner saboteur as well. How many times has that inner voice told you to give up or that something can't be done, only for you to find out that what you believed was going to happen never did?

I recommend that you read *Positive Intelligence* by Shirzad Chamine for more information on this topic.

The power of positive intelligence can lift you to new heights.

Chapter 62

Ice-Cream Socials

Two scoops of vanilla with whipped cream and a cherry on top. Mouthwatering and no calories—not!

As a team, you have been working hard for a common goal, and after months of preparation, you have finally reached the peak. Are you going to perform and succeed or go back to the drawing board to improve?

No matter the outcome, you know your team has worked hard to exceed expectations and is psyched to showcase all their accomplishments. Indeed, the team performed as a great team would.

Now what? How are you going to show your appreciation for their hard work? Is it time to write another thank-you card, or is it time to mix it up?

As the title of this chapter alludes, an ice-cream social is the perfect way to celebrate a team accomplishment. It's simple but very powerful; after all, everybody loves ice cream, and it's even better when served by senior leadership.

Don't screw this up by coming up short; nothing is more demoralizing than running out of ice pops.

As a leader, one of the most important things you will ever do is serve ice cream.

Chapter 63

Succession Planning—Are You Ready to Leave?

Have you ever been left at the altar all by yourself or failed to develop a plan B? It's like planning an outdoor party in monsoon season and forgetting to order a tent just in case it rains.

Have you ever worked for a successful manager who was the shining star of the organization? He or she seemed to be involved in everything and was perceived to make improvements that were difficult to attain. He or she was a celebrated success story, going above and beyond until that day he or she left to take that dream job. It only took a few weeks until it all fell apart, leaving others to wonder what happened.

This is not an atypical occurrence when a great doer leaves the organization and has failed to develop the next leaders to take over where he or she left off.

Highly effective leaders start developing the next leaders of the organization on day one and will support them until the day they leave. A true measurement of success is the fact that your business unit runs on without skipping a beat and continues to improve and push performance to another level.

So make a promise to yourself to be a giver from day one; involve up-and-coming leaders in the decision-making processes, and share your deep experiences, both good and bad. Someday, when you are ready to move on, it will be satisfying to know life goes on without skipping a beat.

Succession planning is a badge of honor, especially when it works.

Chapter 64

Good Ol' Boys' Club: Should I Join?

There is no group more famous than the Rat Pack as an example to discuss the good ol' boys' club. The Rats included Sammy Davis Junior, Frank Sinatra, and Dean Martin, just to mention a few. It was the club to belong to back in the day, real or perceived; one needed the blessing of the Rats to get anywhere in the entertainment industry.

Is it any different in your workplace? I bet you know a Rat Pack in your place that holds the unofficial strings to some of the most desired positions, titles, or goodies. All you have to do is sell your soul to the devil and walk the plank!

Are your personal values aligned with this type of back-alley behavior? Are you sure you want to spend endless hours in the bar or on the golf course kissing some ass, hoping for a return on investment?

I know what I will and won't do; this is not an avenue I have gone down, nor do I recommend you do it. It's a world of unknowns, and you are only as good as your last act—especially in a good ol' boys' club.

Instead, pursue a positive, value-based career path by working harder than the next guy, and be in constant pursuit of excellence. If you are not noticed by your current employers, you will be rewarded by either a competitor or knowing you didn't sell your soul down the river.

Be a trendsetter and form an all-inclusive group based on principles of shared learning, coaching, and mentoring. Take the responsibility of guiding the next generation to a path of personal happiness and success, wherever that may be.

Stay true to yourself at all times.

Chapter 65

Fiscal Responsibility

Have you ever had the urge to ask a business manager at your first interview to see his credit-card statements? What would it tell you about the person? If he or she can't manage a personal checkbook, how would he or she manage mine?

Everybody says they are fiscally responsible. Does this really mean you spent only what you have in your budget, or is it underspending by 10 percent or even overspending by 10 percent?

Fiscal responsibility for leaders on any level should mean you are thoughtful about *what* you spend, *where* you spend, and *when* you spend it. There's a right time to spend, save, or reduce wasteful spending. It all depends on the business cycle you are in.

Fiscal responsibility means understanding and appreciating the larger picture of your environment, including long-term needs and short-term constraints. One needs to be proactive and stay ahead of the curve before it is too late. Cost cutting is always painful and disruptive; however, a fiscally responsible manager would have planned for a rainy day already, thereby minimizing impact on morale and ability to provide services.

Fiscal responsibility means planning for capital improvements that will yield the highest returns on investment. Being a responsible leader, you will live with the principle of creativity over capital and challenge yourself to make do with what you have before opening your wallet. This is normal for those of us who lack access to cash, but here's a word of caution to those who have the funding necessary to execute: Don't just spend because you can. Do you want it or need it? Know your answer before putting that final approval signature on paper or even making the request for funding.

Make it your job to understand the profit-and-loss cycle.

Chapter 66

Thank-You Cards—When Was the Last Time You Wrote One?

Fewer than 10 percent of you can honestly say you have handwritten a thank-you note for someone who did something spectacular. In fact, I'll bet most of you don't even have thank-you cards in your current inventory.

The computer age is ruining us a little more each day. We are slowly losing touch with reality and sinking deeper into the vortex of the iCloud.

Get your head out of the *clouds* and start behaving like a caring, empathetic human being who still enjoys true penmanship or some actual human interaction rather than hiding behind that keyboard.

How hypocritical of me while I'm banging away on my computer, writing short stories when I should be interacting with those around me. I hope the lessons in my short stories will be a step in the right direction to preserving human relations before it is too late.

Do you know the power of a handwritten thank-you card? Let me tell you, I have written thousands of quick notes of appreciation in e-mails, and 100 percent of them are either deleted or stored in a folder that has not been opened since the message was originally sent. I'm not saying there's no value in the moment, but I'm sure there's very limited long-term value.

The power of the handwritten thank-you card can be seen every time I walk into someone's office. Most people proudly display their cards and are asked about them often, which gives them an opportunity to share. I still have every single handwritten card I have ever received in my desk, and I proudly display the most recent ones *on* my desk.

Five minutes of your time to write a heartfelt thank-you is one of the greatest satisfiers you can ever give your teammates.

Start handwriting thank-you cards today without delay.

Chapter 67

Walk Rounds with Who, Where, and When?

This is another laborious undertaking some brilliant mind in the back office came up with but that has not yet been exposed to the angry wolves on the front lines. Why expose myself to questions about things to which I have no answers?

This is a prime example of old thinking that needs to go down the sewer along with a direct management style. Exemplary leaders of tomorrow need to be committed to spending time with the frontline staff not only to be open to tough questions but also to find opportunities to lead through context, taking their time to explain the why.

All too frequently, frontline staff's top two comments regarding management are associated with the words *respect* and *disconnect*. As leaders, we should take to heart the mandate to spend more time exploring ways to improve both areas of opportunity, and there's no better way to do this than by completing daily walk rounds.

Depending on your current function, identify key stakeholders for your areas of responsibilities or direct reports to commit to scheduled walk rounds as often as necessary. Develop key objectives and share with your staff that you will be rounding on their respective units.

The key message to your staff should include that walk rounds are supportive in nature, not punitive. Staff should feel comfortable to come up and ask questions and make suggestions for improvements.

It's a great time to listen twice as much as you talk, with frequent acknowledgment of staff's dedication to their profession and patients or customers.

Your attitude must be warm, open, teachable, respectful, and in the now.

Chapter 68

Physical Fitness—an Integral Piece of the Puzzle

Do you think your weight, stamina, snoring, chronic diseases, insomnia, alcohol consumption, or smoking has any impact on your ability to be an effective *positude* leader?

Let's go the unscientific route, although there's plenty of evidence that all of the above are potential negative contributors to being effective in life.

Let's assess your own fitness for a minute. Nobody is watching, and there's no need to write anything down—just a moment of pure honesty with yourself.

I fibbed—I was watching and listening. You are right; you should lose those extra ten pounds, improve your sleeping pattern, reduce alcohol consumption to weekends only, and finally, go see your physician for a plan to control any addictions.

Effective leadership requires you to be in equilibrium with the mental, physical, and relationship states of mind. This will require you to carefully map out where you are today and what you can attain within a reasonable period of time. Make yourself the next process-improvement project.

To be very honest, I have been working on each of these vital components and continue to struggle with some more than others. The fact that I'm committed to being a better human physically and mentally allows me to continue to grow as a leader and person. Trust me—it's a work in progress.

This is one of those topics that are deeply personal to the reader and also the most frequently disregarded topic if action is not taken immediately.

To change, be the change you want to see.

Chapter 69

Mental Fitness—an Absolute Must

This place is driving me crazy! I'm pulling my hair out every step of the way. I'm banging my head against the wall out of frustration. I feel like I work in a nuthouse. What's Einstein's definition of insanity?

We all can relate to any of the above. But the real questions remain: How do you deal with stresses both at work and at home? Are you mentally fit to deal with adversity? Do you have a mechanism to debrief or discuss your feelings? Do you maintain a regimen on a regular basis to preserve your sanity?

As leaders, we tend to be alpha personalities who want to exceed in every task and function, which elevates our stress levels into the stratosphere. Sadly, most don't realize or appreciate the long-term impact on our physical well-being.

Let's concentrate on your mental fitness and ways to stay sane. It's no different from going to the gym to work on your six-pack; if you don't put in the time, you will not get the results you desire.

Mental fitness should become a top priority for you, especially if you are transitioning from a frontline position into management or from being in charge of a department to being the top dog in the organization.

First, recognize what has a calming effect on you. It's different for each of us—no cookie-cutter suggestions here. Meditation, sports events, playing cards, seeing a psychologist or counselor—what is most important is for you to find the sweet spot where you can debrief, deflate, let go, and regroup. We all need a safe place, whether a religious institution, golf course, or gym. You need to make it a priority for yourself to stay in optimum mental fitness to be truly effective as a leader.

Personally, I choose to meditate daily, even if it is just for a minute or two.

Chapter 70

Being Awesome

Did you awaken this morning deciding you were going to do more of the same or finally take a definitive step toward being awesome?

Going through every day knowing the outcomes or, at best, marginally contributing is just not for me. I decided some time ago that I wanted to make a difference and needed to be the change I wanted to see. No, I'm not talking about being a king or even wanting to be the boss. I want to make a difference by simply greeting everyday people with a heartfelt "Good morning—have a wonderful day!"

Today, I must say it at least a hundred times a morning, bringing smiles to some somber faces along the way. Actually, some try to beat me to the punch now and say it before I can. My behavior is having an impact; I'm getting my desired results through a simple change in my personal culture. Can you imagine what we could do if each of us makes a positive change and sticks to it until it becomes the new norm?

Results come from our actions, which are based on our beliefs and deep, personal experiences. The question remains: Are you satisfied with your results?

Honestly, most of us can use a bit more *positude* in our lives and need to shift our results, actions, and beliefs. Set a challenge for yourself to be simply awesome.

Awesomeness is an outward expression that can be seen, felt, and experienced in everything you do. Be awesome not just for you but for the responses you will generate and the happiness it creates, however brief it is.

Awaken tomorrow morning and take a definitive step toward awesomeness.

Chapter 71

Why Mentoring Is Important to Personal Growth

Would you ever consider climbing Mount Everest without a guide? Unless you don't like yourself or have no intention to make it off the mountain, you would, of course, seek mentorship from those who have gone before you.

Well, why would you try to figure out how to be a great leader without seeking advice from the very best and brightest in your industry? Great mentors can make the difference in reaching your long-term goals or not. I put great emphasis on the plural *mentors*, as each brings something else to the table. It takes a village to get you to the top.

Where to start? First, make sure you are teachable. Are you ready to seek advice and critical feedback? Are you ready to act upon advice? Only once you are ready to learn should you proceed.

Although convenient, your mentor doesn't need to be someone in your immediate work group or even institution. I have had mentors both within and outside my organization; each brought a different perspective.

Don't look at mentors to give you or search for your next job; separate the two completely. A mentor/mentee relationship is built over a period of time.

As an aspiring leader, you need to continuously stay on a path of self-discovery by reading a lot, joining professional organizations, and spending time giving back to others by being a mentor.

Mentorship is about personal and professional growth, not career advancement.

Chapter 72

How to Be a Great Mentee

Are you ready to build your next long-term relationship with someone other than your spouse? Becoming a mentee or being a mentor can be a lifelong commitment—of course, amicable divorces are possible.

Being a great mentee means understanding your role in the relationship. As a mentee, you are not the subordinate but a partner in a personal, trusting, learning relationship. However, great mentees are the ones to take the initiative, follow up, and follow through on commitments made. A great mentee is highly motivated to learn and expand his or her professional knowledge to the next level.

Start by answering the question, "Why do you want to be mentored?" Do you understand the fiduciary relationship between mentor and mentee? Do you understand that this relationship is built on respect and clarity?

If you are truly committed and ready to be mentored, take the first step to make contact with someone you would model yourself after or someone who is a role model in the industry. Approach the initial meeting not as a job interview but rather as a professional networking meeting with the intent of asking to be mentored and providing reasons why you have chosen him or her.

Always be prepared for each session; bring talking points, but be nimble in your discussion. There's not one good way to be mentored; however, usually the mentee will ask lots of questions and describe scenarios, whereby the mentor provides guidance that should challenge your thinking process. Be a great listener.

Having a big brother or sister is a powerful tool in your armament.

Chapter 73

Professional Associations—Should I Join?

As a *positude* leader, you have made a pledge to both your staff and your boss that you are committed to the position and everything that comes with it, including developing short-term and long-term strategies.

Those who take the time to manage only from within, disregarding all external information or knowledge, will be less effective. Over time, they will fail to keep up with the standards. Dedicated time should be set aside to read, watch, or listen to your peers across the spectrum. The easiest and least expensive way to stay in touch with best practices is to belong to professional associations.

One should look forward to monthly publications filled to the brim with information and trials that were completed on their dime. It's your time to sort through the information and only take what you think is worth trialing.

Don't just belong to a professional association; actually get involved, give back, and contribute. Sharing is like receiving; teaching is a form of learning.

Turn your Washingtons into Hamiltons by utilizing information shared.

Set the bar high for your staff and encourage them to follow your lead by joining relevant professional associations and publications. Pay it forward by covering first-year subscription costs.

Being the best takes the best information.

Chapter 74

Hiring: Passion, Skills, Knowledge, and Ability

Think back to your absolute worst hire in your career. What happened? Did you see something during the interview that disappeared when the person came to work? Did you fall in love with that candidate's knowledge and ability to articulate complex issues, only to find the person failed to translate knowledge into ability to share and inspire? Or perhaps you took the time to test his or her ability, just to learn it was skin-deep at best.

More often than not, you failed to assess his or her true passion for the job!

I'm pretty sure that any of the above will ring true for one hire or another; however, I'm 100 percent sure that lack of passion was the most likely reason.

How do you go forward and not make the same mistake twice? You should assess your own passion first. Do you still have what it takes to get the job done? Are you still getting up every morning with a bellyful of fire, ready to make a difference from the moment you enter the parking lot till the time you go home again?

Only if you stare into the mirror and convincingly tell yourself you are passionate and committed can you present yourself with confidence in front of your next potential hire. Passion needs to be felt; it's a two-way street. Your passion will be that of a visionary, someone to believe in and someone to follow.

In return, you can assess the passion of your candidates when they describe their knowledge, skills, and ability. If they can muster up the passion to tell their own stories, how will they tell yours?

My opening question is this: "Please bring your résumé alive in three to five minutes." If they are done in less than a minute, the likelihood that they will be successful is severely limited. Cut your losses when you have the chance; never settle, and never give up on passion.

Chapter 75

When to Let Go

When should you let go? When it's not too late! That's sometimes easier said than done.

Some will say only after the fact that the writing was on the wall, though they generally failed to say anything while the destruction (poor performance or attitude that negatively affects others in the workplace) was taking place. One must question why nobody has the courage to say something before it's too late in these situations.

As a leader, you never want to be in the position of being too late, meaning permanent damage has been done, financial penalty incurred, or customers lost.

Leaders must be on continuous surveillance, looking for signs and symptoms of disruption, incompetence, or overconfidence. This is a steep hill to climb all by yourself; therefore, a great leader will recruit lots of help along the way. These recruits need to be developed into keen observers of certain behaviors and able to intercede in a timely manner.

As I have mentioned before, unless the person you are dealing with is purposely destructive, one should always give benefit of the doubt and duly investigate why such behavior exists. Follow the rules of asking, requesting, telling, and directing as a four-step process to providing supportive redirection to your problematic staff member.

Leave no doubt behind that staff members who are nonresponsive after being directed will need to be let go.

Don't allow a cancer to metastasize.

Chapter 76

Creativity over Capital

Some staffers are like nagging children: never satisfied with what they have and always wanting more—and the more expensive, the better, of course.

What happened to creativity? Do we still think with both sides of the brain? Or are we just stuck in the habit of acquiring rather than creating?

Most of us will need to learn to manage with what we have, not what we want, simply due to the fact that our bank accounts can't support our wants.

Actually, I'm a strong believer that those who have little are the most resourceful and learn to manage with little or nothing at all. They also tend to be more satisfied with the little things in life, both at home and at work.

As a manager, you need to encourage creativity and empower staff to think outside the box. This does not come naturally for most staffers—it's not that they don't want to, but they have not been allowed to do it. Some of this is perception versus actuality; however, perception needs to be countered through empowerment.

You will be amazed how creative staff can be when allowed and what can be done with very limited resources. All you need to do is set the stage.

Creativity allows you to stretch a dollar in many ways; just don't forget to be creative in your own way to acknowledge staff for *their* creative ways of getting the job done.

Encourage your staff to be the change they want to see.

Chapter 77

Labor Relations—Not Again!

My stomach turns just from the thought of having to waste more of my valuable time dealing with belligerent staff members who are clearly not interested in performing, but who are being protected by their union representatives. All of you can relate to this on some level. What a waste!

One should ask, "Did I really do everything possible to recover this staff member. Why did it go this route? Was it me or them?"

By the time one gets an appointment with labor relations, it's likely too late to recover your staff member. Labor relations should have done their due diligence before the initial hearing and ought to be in a great position to be an arbitrator in finding a common solution to a current problem.

As a new leader, I would strongly encourage you to start building strong relationships with your union representatives or unit leaders. Create a safe work environment to conduct bilateral dialogue based upon facts, not hearsay or imagination.

Bring your union leaders to the table and find common understanding and common goals—it's the best remedy to stay away from labor relations.

From time to time, labor relations are a necessary evil for good.

Chapter 78

EQ: It's a Muscle

"I pick it up and put it down!" Imagine a thick Dutch accent to go along with this short quote. Building muscle requires repetitive-motion activities to shape for desired results. Fail to exercise regularly, and you will slip right back from a six-pack to a solid keg!

Emotional quotation, better known as EQ, is not something you are born with. Of course, almost all of us are born and raised to feel some sympathy or be empathetic, but very few of us have ever truly unlocked its capacity.

In the recent past, at a time when direct leadership was still held in high regard, emotional intelligence was not spoken about or even on the radar screen. Fast-forward a few years, and we have changed from Gen X to Gen Y and now the millennials. Direct leadership has been substituted with servant leadership, which requires heavy reliance on your inherent EQ skills.

I would strongly recommend you go online and search for a free EQ test; it will provide some insights to where you fall on the scale and how much work lies ahead of you to build the EQ muscle required to be a highly effective collaborative leader.

There's not one magical way of gaining the EQ required in today's challenging environment; therefore, it is of the utmost importance that you make a long-term commitment to exercising your EQ muscle continuously, seeking feedback or reassessment to ensure you are gaining EQ muscle.

It's a little less about your IQ and a whole lot more about your EQ.

Chapter 79

PQ: Positive Intelligence—Who Made This Up?

Alphabet soup for the brain: IQ, EQ, PQ, BQ. What's next—SQ, for sleeping intelligence? I think I'm on to something and should claim it for myself! Actually, PQ really is worth talking about, because it will set your mind straight to lead from a positive perspective.

Let's get positive. We have been around negative people and find it to be draining and less than stimulating, to say the least. I always wonder why people get stuck in the continuous loop of negativity. Can they break the cycle?

Let's take an unscientific approach to this imprecise science of the brain. We know more about Mars or the bottom of the ocean than we know about the brain.

Truly negative people are in a closed-loop cycle that will generate only negative thought. The glass is half-empty, even when it is full to the top.

Truly positive people spend minimal time on the negative and maximum time on the positive. They will find a way to make dog shit smell like rose petals.

Most of us are somewhere in between, with a tendency to go either positive or negative, depending on the environment we are in—easily influenced by others.

What we need to recognize is that most of us can become positive; however, it takes thirty to ninety days of repetitive actions each day to convert from negative to positive. Challenge yourself and go for it.

Every day when I wake up, no matter the weather, I tell myself why we are fortunate to have rain, snow, ice, sun, wind, and so on.

Chapter 80

Is IQ Still Important?

IQ is so out of date. Who cares how smart you are? Isn't it way more important to know how you *apply* your wisdom? I care more about the person's emotional intelligence and behavioral capacity than knowing he or she has an IQ above 120.

It's that dirty, little, not-so-white lie that is told every time someone asks you if you know your IQ. Truth be told, most people have never taken an actual IQ test, other than a free test online. If you are really smart, you take the test two or three times in a row, until you get the IQ score you wish to publish on your Facebook account.

However, in the real world, we care less about your IQ scores and far more about your passion in or zest for life—without either, you can't unlock your full potential and apply yourself to the best of your abilities.

Instead of someone with a high IQ, I'd rather work with or for or hire someone who possesses the behavioral capacity and emotional aptitude to work with others, such as patients, clients, or other members of the organization. It's not how smart you are; it is how well you can work with others, how well you can inspire others, and how well you can lead others.

My recommendation to those who have relied on their IQs up to this point in time is to test your EQ, PQ, and BQ. If you score low on any of them, sink your teeth into improving them, because you can; these are different from your IQ, which is set at the time of birth.

Be smart and go beyond your IQ.

Chapter 81

What Is Your Behavioral Capacity?

The new kid on the block! Let's start with a simple equation:

$$\text{Performance} = f(\text{Technical Skill})(\text{Behavioral Capacity})$$

(Credit to the master of BQ, Michael Frisina. Google his name and buy his books.)

It is an absolute that we blame much of what goes wrong on our technical skills and spend too much time retraining them; meanwhile, we ignore the root cause, which most likely is due to our low behavioral capacity.

Why do we ignore addressing behavioral issues? Simply because it is difficult to give feedback to our staff. It's against human nature to say something negative or to have that difficult conversation, but continuing on the path of least resistance undoubtedly will cause more harm in the future.

We all need to start with assessing our own behavioral capacity and make necessary adjustments to gain muscle tone in this vital area of *positude* leadership.

The power of behavioral capacity should not be underestimated. Get this right, and you'll see transformation in front of your eyes. Since we tend to ignore this issue most often, those with low BQs are rarely aware. Unlock their magic as well by addressing BQ issues head-on in a safe environment. Feedback is a necessary evil of leadership and really should be seen as your great ally, especially if both your BQ and EQ are in the right hemisphere.

Get this right, and life will be that much easier.

Chapter 82

Are You Accountable to Yourself?

Let's take the sensitive subject of weight management to highlight our intrinsic failure to be accountable to the self. Let's enjoy a pure moment of honesty and admit we have all lied about our weight and understated our total food consumption when measuring for weight loss. I don't care if you're skinny, fat, or somewhere in between; we have all done it. We are way too easy on ourselves, because we can be.

But we are not doing ourselves any favors by being dishonest, regardless of the subject matter.

Let's look at a different angle of the same problem. As a leader, you are making sure your teammates are accountable to the team. If they are not, we should have feedback sessions to address this lack of behavioral capacity. How often do we really follow through and address the lack of accountability? I can tell you from experience that it isn't often enough. Why not? Because we lack the behavioral capacity to have difficult situations and therefore fail to be accountable to the self.

Two different angles—same results. Now what?

The first step is to admit we have a problem with self-accountability and to seek guidance in finding a solid solution.

From deep experience, make a real effort to become self-accountable before you can be accountable to others. Set *SMART* goals for yourself, and carefully measure for success. Be tough on yourself, and have predetermined penalties in place when you fail to deliver. Follow through!

Look in the mirror and stay true to yourself.

Chapter 83

Silence

This is the easiest short section I have written.

(Left intentionally blank)

We have all been on the receiving end of the silent treatment and most likely have given it to somebody else.

Oh, how uncomfortable it is, wondering nervously what it all means and how to react. Some get angry, while others simply disconnect. Regardless of how you feel, the silent treatment stirs up deep emotions, and they're rarely satisfying. However, both the giver and the receiver are contributors to this state of mind.

There's another form of silence that allows one to get into a deeper state of listening. One can pick up sounds and emotions otherwise not heard. This type of silence can bring deep happiness and fulfillment.

Silence is powerful in more ways than one. *Positude* managers should not seek the silent treatment, but they *should* strive for silent surroundings where fewer words are spoken unless they are truly meaningful and on target.

As you grow as a leader, you will find your inner silence and learn to manage silence due to conflict. Silence in conflict, if not managed, will lead to disaster over time. Through quiet observation before intervention, though, one will be more impactful when breaking the silence, allowing a path to healing to emerge.

Superior communication and listening skills will prevent the silent treatment; however, this takes much practice and patience to master.

Silence is sometimes the best noise.

Chapter 84

Ask, Tell, Ask—Do You?

Let's play a little game to set the stage. Randomly place all numbers one through nine on a blank piece of paper. Use the entire paper. Look at it for two seconds. Turn it over, and now recreate what you saw on the reverse.

Strange...I can't see you, but I know you got less than 40 percent right!

What is my point? We are horrible at remembering what we just saw or heard. As humans, we are *so* bad at it that chimpanzees beat us at the same game nine out of ten times.

As a leader, what lesson can you learn from this simple game? If you give verbal instructions to your staff, they most likely will forget 80 percent of what you said before they leave your office—sad but true.

How can you counter this phenomenon? It's time to outsmart the brain by hardwiring your message, using "ask, tell, ask" or motivational-interviewing techniques.

First, make sure you treat each person as an individual. We are wired differently and likely learn in different ways; however, each of us improves performance significantly when we are engaged in the conversation.

Second, make sure the receivers understand your request. Verify by asking them to repeat what you've asked of them. This will give both parties the opportunity to ensure you have a common understanding, and if necessary, clarifications can be made.

Finally, close the conversation by repeating your request. You are now set up for greater success.

Use this technique in every conversation.

Chapter 85

KISS—Keep It Simple, Stupid

It really doesn't matter which topic we talk about or what process we need to improve; we have a natural tendency to overthink, underestimate, and fail to perform simply because we are thinking, speaking, or doing too quickly.

I have been guilty of this too many times. My enthusiasm and passion get the better of me when I can see a solution, particularly when not everybody else can, for whatever reason. Just because I can or have the ability to solve an issue doesn't mean my solution will be successful, especially when it depends on others while I am not around.

Have you ever overpromised and underperformed? Of course you have. Did you learn a lesson for the future, or have you been a multi-occasion offender? Most of us have repeated our mistakes not because of ignorance, but because we want to believe we can deliver.

Somebody I don't particularly care for once said, "To eat an elephant, one must do it one bite at a time." This is a very true statement that should be taken to heart.

I'm not sure who said it first, but *KISS*—Keep It Simple, Stupid—is likely the best lesson one can learn as a leader. Don't overdo it. When developing a new process, apply the *KISS* rule to ensure that those who will be following the new process can repeat it. You are likely to be more successful if you take ten little steps versus one giant leap.

If it ain't KISS or SMART, take a step back...and reapply KISS and SMART.

Chapter 86

Networking for Professional Development

Do I really need to have friends at work? Should I make an effort to get to know peers in my organization? Is it really going to be worth my effort to mingle with folks I don't even know?

These are awesome questions you will need to answer for yourself.

There's a right time for networking; however, professional development should be an ongoing effort. When the time is right, you can start networking for professional development and even career advancement.

A wise man once said to me that it takes nine layers of networking to find the right job, if that's what you are interested in.

Another wise man told me that professional development, networking, being a mentee, and mentoring are crucial cornerstones to success.

Start by networking with your peers within your own work group; get to know them on a different level by facilitating conversations about professional growth and sharing experiences. Most importantly, don't sit back and wait for them to come to you. If necessary, organize something yourself. If you build it, they will come; it really works, especially for free coffee and cookies.

Join a local organization, such as the Lions Club, Knights of Columbus, Rotary, local ACHE chapter, and so on. Relate; don't compare. Go with the flow. Listen and observe. When the time is right, participate.

Have fun while networking.

Chapter 87

Paying It Forward—How, When, Why?

Oprah is the best adviser who rarely follows her own advice. What's your first thought when someone says "Oprah"? *Not another diet or best girlfriend story*...What I remember most is her commitment to paying it forward. I love the concept of paying it forward and do so at least weekly in small ways, such as paying for someone's coffee or lunch. Try it for yourself someday; it really feels great.

However, don't stop there. We are not billionaires like Oprah is, but we have something much better to offer: our lifetime experiences. You have something to offer, not unlike those who offered you support and guidance in the past. Think back for a minute and name a few occasions when you received free advice. Each occurrence is a form of paying it forward.

Let's discuss a couple of basic scenarios in which you can pay it forward in your professional life.

As a new or experienced manager or leader, you most likely have at least a handful of staff members who report to you directly. As a leader, it is your responsibility to identify opportunities to shape the futures of your teammates by sharing your experiences, either as a mentor or, more informally, as a coworker.

Another meaningful way is to pay attention to staffers outside your department who are struggling in low-paying positions but who have the potential to do much more. Take the time to acknowledge them every day and strike up a conversation about their aspirations. Find ways to be supportive, and if they are interested, assist them by supplying information, books, and pathways to opportunities that would not otherwise be available to them.

Pay it forward—ROI to follow.

Chapter 88

Checklist—Wheels Down

Go to the NTSB website for just a few minutes and read a few accident reports concerning general aviation. OK, what did you discover? The vast majority of general aviation accidents occur due to pilot error.

What types of errors? Running out of fuel, landing with the gear up, or failure to check weather conditions prior to departure. These errors could have been prevented had the pilots in command (PIC) used a checklist as is strongly suggested by FAA instructors when they go for their check ride to obtain their pilot's licenses.

What does this mean to me? One could say, "Simple. Almost everything we do in health care, or many other businesses, has predetermined process steps. Once we follow them step-by-step, the outcome is highly predictable, and quality is maintained."

Just think for a moment. Placing a central line or Foley catheter, marking a surgical site, developing a profit/loss statement, or shipping a high-valued item across the country—each of these requires individual process steps. If these are not followed in exact order, one could cause an error. If one follows a set checklist step-by-step, the risk of adverse outcome is decreased tenfold.

Complacency is the killer in most of these circumstances: "I have done this a million times. I don't need a stinking checklist"—until, of course, something unpredictable takes place or a distraction occurs. Then mostly preventable errors will, and do, occur.

Don't be a fool; use a checklist.

Chapter 89

Leading Edge versus Trailing Edge

How excited will your staff be when you install a pay phone or a VHS recorder? They will laugh out loud and think you have gone off the deep end!

Staying with the analogy of flying an airplane, hopefully the plane you are flying has two wings, with one on each side of the fuselage. More importantly, look at one of those wings, and what do you see? A leading edge and a trailing edge, far behind.

As a leader, it is your responsibility to carve out enough time to stay on the leading edge of information, best practices, and technology.

If you find yourself on the trailing edge in your current state, devise a plan to get you moving toward the leading edge. Keep a realistic perspective and timeline to prevent frustration and burnout.

Failure to recognize or failure to act will lead to greater inefficiencies and eventually loss of market share.

Working in a capital-poor environment makes staying on the leading edge a greater challenge, but it's not impossible. Concentrate on working within your circle of influence.

If you say you don't have the time, make the time. As a leader, at minimum 10 percent of your time should be dedicated to the future. Look ahead; stay ahead.

Leading-edge behavior leads to innovation and breakthrough.

Chapter 90

When to Pick Up the Phone versus E-mail

Do you remember the telephone extensions of your direct reports? It all depends on your generation: 95+ percent of Gen Xers know them without hesitation. For Gen Yers and millennials, however, there's not a chance in the world they know more than just a few.

Not only are we completely spoiled by autodial, we simply don't pick up the phone to discuss an issue any longer. Texts and e-mail can be sent from your phone from anywhere at any time; however, are these messages as effective as a phone call?

You can argue this issue until the cows come home, but it's undeniable that we hide behind the impersonal text and e-mail because we lack the capacity to address difficult issues head-on. I will be very honest and tell you that texting is a powerful way to tell someone something without interruption; just be mindful that your words are without emotion and can and will be received and interpreted as such.

My boss, a typical Gen-Xer kind of guy, gave me some solid advice a long time ago: live by the rule that if more than three exchanges via e-mail are needed to get the point across, stop, pick up the phone, and finish the conversation.

As a leader, you will be CCed on many e-mails. If you see this behavior from your staff members, simply "reply all" with this message: *Time to pick up a phone.*

Bring emotion and feeling to vital conversations by picking up the phone or walking to one's office to connect face-to-face.

Chapter 91

Creating a Safe Zone

I bet you a dollar that each of you has experienced a similar moment that will stick with you forever—that dreaded call from a heavy-handed HR director with a directive to come to his or her office immediately without further explanation as to why.

I don't care if you are Mr. or Ms. Perfect; your palms will be sweaty, and you will be wondering, *What the hell did I do?* or *Who said what that warrants this directive?*

Would you feel that you are walking into a safe zone? I don't think so, and I'm pretty sure you would agree. Now, don't repeat others' mistakes by doing this to your staff members. An innocent call for assistance can and will be interpreted as an "oh no" moment, which is uncomfortable and unnecessary, to say the least.

Be hyperaware of this, especially when you are starting a new management role. You are setting the stage and want to make a great first impression.

Let's make a promise to create safe zones for your staff members to reduce anxiety levels, which, in turn, will promote transparency and collaboration.

Even a negative feedback session should be done in a safe zone and, if possible, away from your office to create a more neutral zone. Besides, effective managers will have an ongoing dialogue with their direct reports, and there should be no surprises for either, unless, of course, it's something out of left field. Trust me—I have tried just about everything, from meetings in my office to conference rooms. Nothing works as well as going to their offices for a discussion or just a weekly check-in to keep everybody informed.

Be aware, be astute, and be safe.

Chapter 92

Leading with Confident Humility

You catch more flies with honey than with vinegar. Who has not worked for a yeller or a "do this, do that" kind of manager? Ugh, I have come across some of them and have found each one to be less competent than the next one. Is that always true?

Who is that guy who started Apple Inc.? Steve Jobs, right? He was a leader with little humility, who at times was outright abusive to his coworkers, board members, and shareholders alike. Steve Jobs was by all means extremely successful by many measures, so we can say *some* get more with vinegar than honey.

However, confident humility is the preferred choice of leadership, especially in today's workplace and with millennials. Collaboration, sharing, confidence, humility, coaching, and mentoring are the attributes most desired in health care especially.

Becoming a leader with these attributes doesn't come overnight, nor can it be bought off the shelf. It takes hard work, dedication, passion, and proper guidance to acquire the right mix of leadership skills, knowledge, and ability.

Leading with confident humility is a journey of learning, adjusting, and making the most of the mistakes you will inevitably make along the way.

I recommend that you read *Good to Great* by Jim Collins, as he will outline a process to become a level-V leader, which is based on a foundation of confident humility. Take your first step right now; go to www.amazon.com and place your order.

Great leaders are truly teachable.

Chapter 93

Why Be a Servant Leader?

In today's environment, directive leaders, even those who are very nice, are much less accepted than those who choose to lead as servants.

The word *servant* is frequently linked to the word *collaborative*; however, each attribute has a distinctive, different function in effective leadership.

Let's briefly review the differences in style between *directive* and *servant* first.

Directive leaders will interpret a demand and tell staff what to do, when to do it, and how to do it—if they know. At minimum, they will give staff a mandate and a deadline without much discussion. Directive leaders are not necessarily micromanagers; however, they will take that route if necessary.

Servant leaders will interpret new mandates and, before rolling out new processes, will present them to the staff at large, assuming the role of coach, mentor, and remover of barriers of success.

Collaborative servant leaders will bring folks from across the organization together and carefully outline requests through context. They will lead a collaborative effort to find a common understanding and common goals to a sensible solution.

Servant leaders will be able to engage staff on all levels of the organization merely because they show great mutual respect and teachability and tend to be excellent listeners. Servant leaders will seek continuous input and feel a great sense of accomplishment when teams work together in a collaborative manner.

Humility, servant, and collaborative—the gold standard of leadership.

Chapter 94

Keeping a Scorecard

Who wants to shoot some more darts in the dark? First one to twenty points wins. Anybody interested? I doubt it. Anybody feel motivated? I doubt it. Anybody feel a sense of accomplishment? I doubt it.

"We are all working so hard, but for what?" one could say. At least in health care, especially at the bedside, one can see the outcome of the countermeasures, also known as treatment plans. However, go to the back office or frontline registrars; they frequently don't really know how they contribute to the bottom line.

As a leader, do you know what *you* contribute to the bottom line? Most of you don't really measure your performance unless, of course, it's part of your incentive package. The question is: Should you know how you are performing?

I would argue that it's better to know how you are performing against either a baseline measure or an established industry benchmark. We are driven by outcomes and are competitive by nature. It's been part of us since Little League T-ball in first grade. Our scorecard at that time was the scoreboard in the outfield.

I'm strongly suggesting that everybody establishes goals and benchmarks for themselves at the beginning of each calendar or fiscal year. It really should be part of your annual-evaluation process, but we all know what happens to those for the next 364 days after signing your latest performance evaluation.

Maintain a simple scorecard on your desktop, with a handful of driver and outcome metrics that truly matter and align with your personal goals. Be tough on yourself when establishing *red*, *yellow*, and *green* zones for each metric. Use SMART metrics and stretch the goal just far enough that you feel a sense of urgency and difficulty in reaching the green zone.

Chapter 95

Are You on Track?

I'm assuming you followed my advice immediately and have established a well-defined scorecard with meaningful metrics. At a glance, you can tell me what's going right. As much as I'd love to believe that, I know most of you probably are still not convinced about the concept of personalized scorecards.

Let's look at it from a different angle.

You are attending a meeting when suddenly someone asks if your project is on track. *Oh, no, what do I say? Should I just tell a white lie that all is well, or do I ask for a reprieve till the next meeting to make an accurate assessment of progress made?*

You should not wait for someone to ask that question; as a leader, you should want to know how well you are doing at all times—maybe not up to the minute, but you should reassess your progress weekly at least, and most metrics should be maintained on your scorecard.

Knowing the answer to the question will allow you to maintain a sense of urgency, reduce variability, and celebrate successes when benchmarks and goals are met. I would suggest you take some time to get this right. Both keeping the scorecard and tracking your progress over time will create accountability to yourself and your team as a whole. My teams maintain weekly scorecards as I do for myself. Each scorecard is reviewed on a weekly basis from a standpoint of providing supportive servant leadership, coaching, and mentoring opportunities.

The lesson I learned along the way reaffirmed the importance of allowing staff members to select their own personalized performance metrics after carefully outlining performance expectations from a particular work unit in alignment with mission and strategies of the company at large.

Knowing how you are performing on a continuous basis is essential to getting ahead.

Chapter 96

When to Say, "What?"

Let's take a quick look down memory lane. When you were in school, do you remember that kid who always had either an answer or another question? I know we have all experienced this. There are truly stupid questions—or at least untimely comments—particularly those that come at 5:00 p.m. on a Friday, when everybody wants to go home to their families or, for our single readers, to happy hour to look for love.

My boss once said, "Less is more." Take that advice as you go forward. One of my professors told me, "Every word must mean something." This is especially true when developing a PowerPoint presentation.

Some of us have the gift of gab, and others don't, but one commonality that exists among all great leaders is their listening skills. When you listen, you can't talk.

Another golden rule to live by is the ability to keep conversations confidential. This is much harder than you may think—there are lots of little ears around you at all times. Be mindful when, where, and to whom you are speaking. I have been the victim of eavesdropping on several occasions. It doesn't feel good; however, it is a leader's responsibility to maintain integrity of information, so be aware.

I would also suggest that you use your intuition. Before you say or write anything, listen to that inner voice. When in doubt, hold off on pushing the send button or speaking in public. Verify with your coach, mentor, or boss before proceeding. Unlike an e-mail, what you say can't be erased or pulled back.

Situational awareness will save your butt.

Chapter 97

Patient Experience Should Come First

Let's make a deal: patients = anyone paying for a service at your hospital.

At some point in time, our customers will be our patients. Regardless, it should be our mission to put our patients at the center of our existence if we truly are to succeed.

What does it really mean to put our patients first? What is more important, or what is most important? We can all agree that safety and quality must be our top priorities in health care. Timeliness, satisfaction, and respect are close seconds.

Patient experience is a mind-set more than a technical skill. We can certainly learn new techniques; however, our willingness to put patient experience above our own needs is a behavioral choice. All too frequently, we find managers, directors, executives, and frontline staff doing what is good for them and not so much for our patients. This can't be tolerated, and as managers or even coworkers, we need to point this behavior out to offenders and hold them accountable for having the right behaviors.

As a manager, you have to enter the building in the right frame of mind. Not unlike at Disney, every single encounter with our internal and external customer counts. You are on display all the time. At Disney, you would be considered a stage character on live TV.

This simply means you have to live the behaviors you seek from your staff. You will fail at times, which is only natural. Recognize it—don't make excuses; apologize, and start anew.

If you don't see yourself in this role or can't find it in yourself to address bad behaviors, you might not be the right person for the job. Maybe you are burned out or too distracted with personal issues.

Chapter 98

Should We Compare or Relate?

It's time for a deep, personal experience that taught me a lesson for life.

I immigrated to the United States in 1988 as an eighteen-year-old confused young man running from my own demons and searching for a new solution, only to find more of the same enabling hoodlums who continued to feed my addictions to negative attention, alcohol, and aggression.

Only by the grace of God did I make it through a rough couple of years with lots of support along the way. There were lots of enablers, but I also met those who were willing to speak the truth. What saved me is the fact that I always worked harder than the next guy and was afforded opportunities that otherwise would not have existed. That is still the truth today.

In 1989, I met a man named Danny, a recovering alcoholic and drug addict himself, who used his personal experiences to become a certified alcohol-addiction counselor. He owned a small bar and restaurant in upstate New York. "Kind of strange," you might say. "A recovering alcoholic who owns a bar." But he still had to make a living until that time when he built up a new client base and was able to sell his beloved possession.

Danny did me two big favors in life. First, he invited me to live and work with his family, and, second, he showed me a better way of living without the use of alcohol.

On June 6, 1989, Danny took me to a youth Alcoholics Anonymous meeting in Binghamton, New York. He gave me a simple instruction: "Shut up, sit down, and relate; don't compare." Sixty minutes later, I learned about myself what I had been searching for, and I quit drinking that day and ever since.

To feel the plight of your patients, relate; don't compare. Empathy is relating, understanding, appreciating, and respecting what your patient is feeling.

Chapter 99

Team Concord—Do You Have It?

When you see a sports team leave its locker room on the way to their field of play, what do they often do?

Just before they leave, they recite a team song, phrase, or quotation or slap a sign above the door, calling for unity, power, energy, strength, wisdom, encouragement, or something similar. It is something that brings the teammates together before they go into battle.

Health care and business are no different; we need to be on top of our game at all times, because the impact of our mistakes could lead to injury and even death. Although some hospitals have instituted morning safety huddles, most have not yet followed this trend.

Why wait for someone to tell you that you have to do it? Do it because it's the right thing to do.

Bring your team together and request they create a short power statement that signifies the type of service they want to provide to their patients or customers. Start by putting key attributes—such as *safety, quality, service excellence, patient experience*, and the like—on paper. There's always someone on the team who is a creative writer and can glue it all together.

Take pride in your team by posting this power statement prominently in your unit, and recite it at every huddle.

Team concord creates team unity.

Chapter 100

Personal Elevator Speech: You Have Thirty Seconds...Go!

Let's pretend for a moment: You are the rising star in your organization but have not yet reached the level where you have regular interactions with your CEO. You are on the tenth floor on your way to the cafeteria to pick up your second, much-needed cup of coffee. You are all by yourself; the elevator stops on the ninth floor, and your CEO walks in. He's a friendly fella and recognizes you from a project you recently presented at one of the hospital-wide forums.

The big moment has arrived; he greets you and asks you how you are doing and what is keeping you busy these days. Panic sets in, your mouth dries up, you are staring at the floor, and before you get anything truly comprehensible out of your mouth, the elevator arrives at the second-floor executive suites, and out steps your CEO with a friendly good-bye, encouraging you to keep up the great work you are doing.

Oh no, what just happened? It's all a complete blur. Why was I not able to articulate what I'm working on or what barriers stand in the way of our success? Was it stage fright or being unprepared?

Unprepared it was—with a little stage fright to top it off!

Learn a valuable lesson from those who have been there before you. Today, start writing down short, well-rehearsed talking points that will describe your current project, your professional accomplishments, your professional goals, barriers to success, vetted business plans, and so on. One size doesn't fit all; you will need to develop several short paragraphs for different scenarios and people.

Don't live with regret. I told you so!

Chapter 101

Finding a Role Model

I want to be just like Prince, the artist, but I don't know how to play a single instrument or even sing. Would Prince be a great role model for me as a hospital administrator?

As usual, you can argue everything from different sides of the equation. Prince might be a great role model, because he learned through hard work how to play twenty-seven instruments; that's a lesson to me that determination and practice can make you competent in many related areas of practice. On the other hand, living like a hermit is not something desirable in a leader.

If you make an assessment of prominent leaders across the industry, you will find that each has attributes that should be modeled, and it's likely that some characteristics should be skipped over. None of us is perfect—nor are you, just in case you didn't know that. My wife reminds me regularly to continue to search for perfection!

My suggestion would be to carefully observe leaders in action or, if they have gone before you, to read their autobiographies—Jack Welch, Colin Powell, Condoleezza Rice, George Patton, Bill Clinton, John Paul II, and the like. You have so many to choose from, and each has something to give to you—their lessons learned and the solutions that assisted them through difficult times.

It is your job as a leader to find the right balance in your leadership style; there's no cookie-cutter recipe for success. Learn what not to do and learn what to do more of. As you progress through your career, maintain a list of what not to do; it's forgotten too easily, and you don't want to make the same mistakes.

Be all you can be; never forget you are a role model too.

Chapter 102

Learn from Others' Mistakes

A failure is only a failure if we fail to learn from it, right? Therefore, mistakes are opportunities.

Maybe it's a little selfish to say, but I prefer to learn from others' mistakes versus my own. To be successful, you can't fear failure. Doing so will leave you paralyzed and doomed to either fail or just be another worker. There's nothing wrong with that, of course, if that's what makes you happy.

Be vigilant in your observation of others. Watch how people prepare, organize, conduct meetings, assign tasks, collect and analyze data, draw conclusions, communicate with key stakeholders and frontline staff alike, implement new processes, and take countermeasures or celebrate successes. You can learn a tremendous amount just through observation of people.

As a former flight paramedic, I have been in some stressful situations and have seen folks make crucial mistakes along the way—none of them because they meant to do harm—due to lack of preparedness, ineffective communications, and lack of teamwork. I have also seen the direct opposite, where partners worked together like a hand in a glove and few words needed to be exchanged to get the best possible outcomes.

Every scenario or action has a potential failure point, especially if there's no backup plan or even a backup to the backup plan. As a leader, you can learn from these mistakes, create opportunities to improve, and prevent the same mistakes from taking place once again.

Be observant and self-aware. It's perfectly OK to make mistakes; however, it's not OK to fail to learn from your mistakes.

From mistakes one can create successes.

Chapter 103

Partnerships Are Vital to Your Success

Don't underestimate the true power of a highly functional partnership. When was the last time you took the time to assess your relationships and partnerships? Maybe you never have or don't know how. One must first understand the value of partnerships by outlining the type of partnership needed to be highly functional.

Not every relationship needs to be truly synergistic, but it must be functional. Take some time to think. Get a piece of paper and put a dot in the middle; that's representative of you. Now add names around you of people you work with, work for, or supervise.

Next, assess the levels of relationships you have with each today. Be truthful; don't sugarcoat anything. This should be a confidential exercise. Now that you know where you are, the real question is this: What type of relationship do you need to have with one another?

Close the gap between current and future states by taking systematic steps to building and nourishing your new relationships. Pay close attention to your partners' intrinsic values; cater to them, as it will strengthen the bond and create a new beginning to excel.

You owe it to yourself to make time for partnership building.

Partnerships are a winning ingredient.

Chapter 104

Closing the Deal

I have written my hundred stories and will finish on my self-imposed deadline of June 1, 2016. It's time to close the deal with one last power story. It should be strong and powerful enough to be seared into your memory.

I sincerely hope some of my experiences will prevent you from making some of the same mistakes or will help you use the tools outlined to set you up for long-term success, professional growth, and *positude* leadership.

However, I skipped over one topic, which is closing the deal on your next professional endeavor or promotion. I have been delaying it because it is my weak point. I can sell you and fight for you; however, when it comes down to *me*, I'm weak and settle too easily.

I have gained strength over time, but I am still not in the right position of power, due to lack of confidence—and maybe just because I'm a nice guy. There's some truth to the statement that nice guys finish last. However, I'm aware of my weakness and am trying to gain strength through my coach, mentor, and my many role models.

I recommend you read *The Art of the Deal* and *The Art of War*; both will put you in a better position for negotiation and understanding the underlying currents in play when making a deal, fighting a war, or getting the right compensation package.

The most important takeaways are that you need to understand your opponent (enemy or hiring agent) and what your bottom line is. Start reasonably high and make the deal above your bottom line, or be prepared to walk away. This is my area of weakness—always suffering from the fear of the unknown.

After confusion comes clarity. Make the deal through clarity.

Chapter 105

Conclusion

Assuming that you took my advice to heart, by relating rather than comparing, I'm sure you were able to recognize yourself in many of the stories. My stories are not unique; however, I approach the solutions a bit differently from most leaders of today.

Utilizing your newly acquired strategies and skills, approach each scenario with a *positude* frame of mind. Believe in yourself, your talented staff, and the other supporting cast members. Be aware of your own mindfulness and that of others. Each scenario requires you to use different skills. It is essential to treat each person as an individual, and as a leader, it is your duty to understand their intrinsic needs.

Be humble in your style, listen more than you talk, be available, encourage, celebrate, and be crystal clear in your vision of expectations.

Together we can do more; one is not better than the other. Each of us has a role to play. As *positude* leaders, it is our role to unlock the potential in each team member and optimize outcomes for those we serve.

Leave this handbook on your desk. Refer to it before you make any major changes to ensure they're aligned with our four strategies and five essential skills for *positude* leadership.

Appendix A: Recommended Reading List

A Sense of Urgency, by John P. Kotter

Change the Culture, Change the Game, by Roger Connors

Good to Great, by Jim Collins

Influential Leadership: Change Your Behavior, Change Your Organization, Change Health Care, by Michael Frisina

Minute Manager, by Ken Blanchard and Spencer Johnson

Our Iceberg Is Melting, by John P. Kotter

Positive Intelligence, by Shirzad Chamine

The Great Employee Handbook, by Quint Studer

The 7 Habits of Highly Effective People, by Stephen Covey

Appendix B:

Reference Materials

Go to www.positudeleadership.com and send me an inquiry for additional information included but not limited to topics below:

Forms Tab

Change Model

Nine-Dot Quiz

Creating a Mini-culture of Excellence

Feedback Model

One-, Three-, and Five-Year Personal-Goals Model

Meeting in the Dark

Blind, Mute, and Distracted

Scorecard

Appendix C:

Tool Kit Expanded Exercises

Step 1	Step 2		Step 3	Step 4	
Name	Determine Level of Partnership		Status Build, Maintain, Repair, Distance	Next Steps	
	Current	Desired		Plan	Completion Date

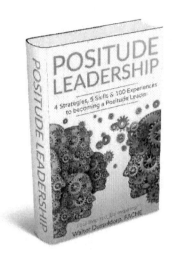

Surviving as a manager in the ever-changing landscape of health care has never been more complicated than today. *Positude Leadership* provides the foundation on which one can be a successful leader and overcome almost any obstacle and, most importantly, create strong bonds with your frontline staff.

—Mark Smith, printshop coordinator

Positude Leadership is a practical how-to guide for tapping into your natural leadership talents, skills, and abilities. Through the lens of Walter Dusseldorp, who focuses high-performance organizations on individual- and team-behavioral capacity, you will learn simple lessons and practices to flourish in your personal and professional growth. Understanding how you can have a positive impact on everyone you encounter, every day, through every interaction, can unleash your leadership potential and touch the lives and careers of those within your sphere of influence.

—Lee Saviola, MS, DO, professional coach

Made in the USA
Columbia, SC
28 April 2018